Physical Therapy in Craniomandibular Disorders

Physical Therapy in Craniomandibular Disorders

Tore L. Hansson, DDS, Odont Dr
Director, Clinic for Craniomandibular Disorders and Facial Pain
St Joseph's Hospital and Medical Center
Phoenix, Arizona

Catherine A. Christensen Minor, PT
Resource Specialist, Outpatient Physical Therapy
St Joseph's Hospital and Medical Center
Phoenix, Arizona

Deborah L. Wagnon Taylor, PT
Manager, Outpatient Rehabilitation Services
St Joseph's Hospital and Medical Center
Phoenix, Arizona

quintessence books

Quintessence Publishing Co, Inc
Chicago, Berlin, London, Tokyo, São Paulo, Moscow

Library of Congress Cataloging-in-Publication Data

Hansson, Tore.
Physical therapy in craniomandibular disorders / Tore L. Hansson, Catherine A. Christensen Minor, Deborah L. Taylor.
p. cm.
Includes bibliographical references.
ISBN 0-86715-192-7
1. Temporomandibular joint—Abormalities—Physical therapy.
2. Temporomandibular joint—Diseases—Physical Therapy.
I. Minor, Catherine A. Christensen. II. Taylor, Deborah L. Wagnon.
III. Title.
[DNLM: 1. Physical therapy—methods. 2. Temporomandibular Joint Diseases—therapy. WU 140 H251p]
RK470.H36 1992
617.5'22—dc20
DNLM/DLC
for Library of Congress 92-1717

quintessence books

Book Designer: Jennifer A. Sabella
Editor: Carol L. Rose
Printing and binding: Ringier America, New Berlin, WI
Printed in USA

Contents

Preface

This book is to be looked upon as a practical guide for physical therapists and dentists who are engaged in the field of craniomandibular disorders and who strive to provide treatment using a team approach. Because this book is not intended to be a textbook, references are kept to a minimum. Above all, this book attempts to initiate standardized care in order to differentiate treatment, to increase the exchange of ideas, and to reduce the incidence of unnecessary treatment.

Our sincere thanks go to our patients who willingly permitted us to use them for demonstration, to Louis Friedman for his initial support, to Terry Gonzalez and Larry Repp for their flexibility and expertise in photography, and to Geri McCorkle for her never-failing enthusiasm in assisting and typing.

Introduction

1

In the management of specific diseases of craniomandibular disorders (CMD), physical therapy (PT) is increasingly important (Kraus, 1988; Antoniotti and Rocabado, 1990). However, often in general practice the patient is exposed to many different randomly chosen modalities, especially when a preliminary diagnosis is lacking.

No direct blame should be placed on the physical therapists, who many times have very little information on the diagnostics and treatment of CMD in their basic education. Their existing knowledge is based upon verbal presentations of short lectures or courses with slide presentations as the only practical source. Although comprehensive literature exists, it is difficult to convert it to practical use. Thorough descriptions of modalities are presented but the specific applications for treating different diagnoses are not given. Another reason for the confusion in daily practice could be the result of the variety of philosophies of the managing dentist. The physical therapist tries his or her best according to the subjective interpretation from the dentist. Traditionally, dentists have not been exposed to PT and do not understand what therapists can do to assist their CMD patients.

Based upon our clinical experience with respect to the most frequently seen conditions, we decided to design this book as a practical guide that will help standardize the management of CMD, familiarize the reader with its treatment, and stimulate research into CMD. We hope to alleviate the confusion shared by many patients and therapists. The duration and intensity of PT will decrease and the outcome results from PT will increase.

In 1980, Hansson et al introduced a concept to primarily distinguish two basic origins of pain, myogenous and arthrogenous, in the stomatognathic system. They applied orthopedic tests of end feel and joint play as well as dynamic and static joint-muscle tests described earlier by Kaltenborn (1974) and Janda (1976). Naeije and Hansson (1986) used these criteria to separate the patients in an electromyographic evaluation of CMD. They found a substantial difference in muscular strength between the two groups of patients. Patients with arthrogenous components to their pain exhibited much weaker muscles than did those patients with myogenous sources of pain. Patients with a myogenous origin of pain were spread over a wider spectrum regarding muscle strength. They were frequently found to have the equivalent strength of the healthy subjects who were used as a control group.

In 1985, Hansson et al thoroughly described the clinical examination of the stomatognathic system. The findings of such an examination should conclude with a preliminary diagnosis. Several clinical studies have been performed using the Hansson et al technique (Bezuur et al 1988a; 1988b; 1989a; 1989b), and from these studies the following general conclusions can be made. Patients suffering from myogenous origins of pain are younger. They show more temporomandibular joint (TMJ) clicking and less TMJ crepitation and the mouth opening is less affected in these patients. The amount of deviation on opening is also smaller, and condylar hard tissue changes are less frequent. However, the vertical condylar asymmetry, calculated from a panoramic radiograph, is greater. In other words, there is more often a morphological difference in vertical dimension between the two TMJ condyles (page 11). In other studies by Schokker et al (1989; 1990a; 1990b) it was found that patients with frequent headaches and myogenous origin of pain more often showed a distance of 5 mm end feel or more. They also exhibited more chronic pain and cervical involvement.

Poor body and head posture seems to be a common link between patients who need PT. A simple way to clinically recognize such a condition (other than by pure observation) is to examine the movements of the cervical spine at the first visit to the dentist by having the patient sit upright in the dental chair without head support. This is advised after the examination of the mandibular movements and joint and muscle functions (see page 12). Usually the findings of such an examination have already been suspected at the preliminary general inspection or during the clinical interview when the patient unconsciously reveals his or her habitual or "normal" facial and body behavior (see page 13). By observing the mandibular movements during the interview, the clinician can likely explain the clinically registered unequal dental wear of the anterior teeth (see page 13). The registration of such movements and dental wear most often directs the examiner to the bruxoposition, which is the trigger for the adverse loading of the stomatognathic system. The general condition of the muscles and ligaments is also frequently revealed by the rest posture of the hands, the feet, and the head of the patient (see page 14). Hyperlaxity of such parts makes the patient rest the particular joint in its border position. Extremely awkward border positions are therefore regularly observed in the whole body (see pages 14 and 15). The lack of muscular tone is frequently obvious from the observation by the dentist, also indicating an immediate referral for a more thorough examination by the physical therapist (see page 15).

Clinical Observations

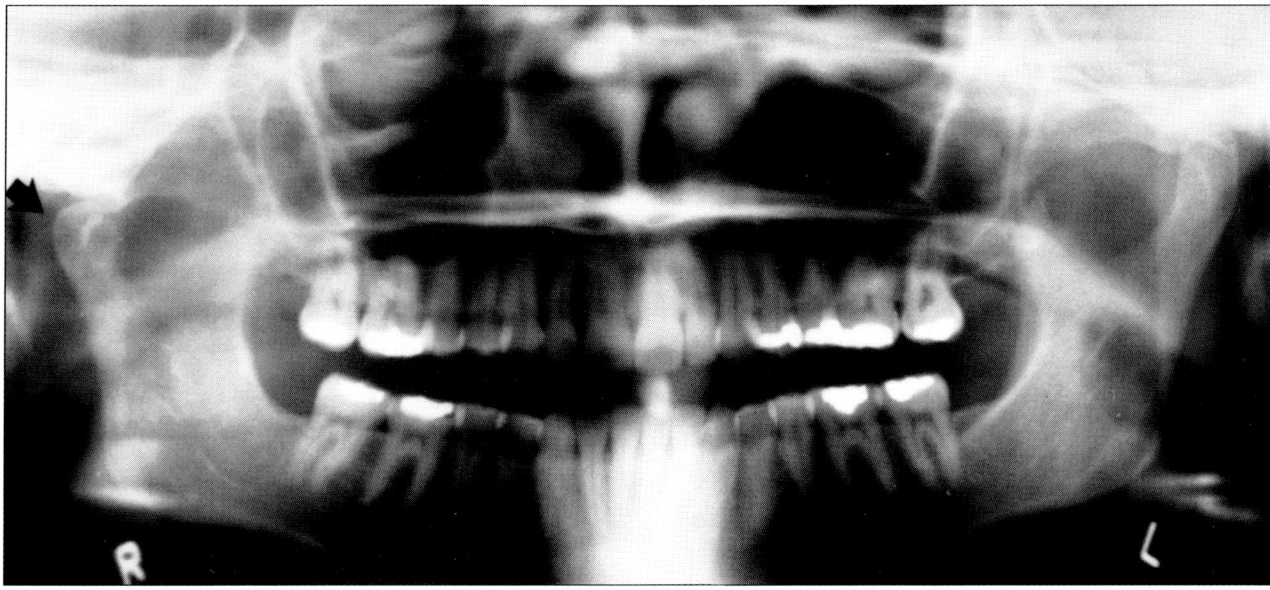

Panoramic radiograph shows the vertical dimension of the right mandibular condyle and ramus to be smaller (shorter) than the left-side dimensions.

EXAMINATION

inspection during rest:

general
specific
asymmetry

inspection during movements:

vertical overbite: mm

mouth opening / closing
deviation (mm)

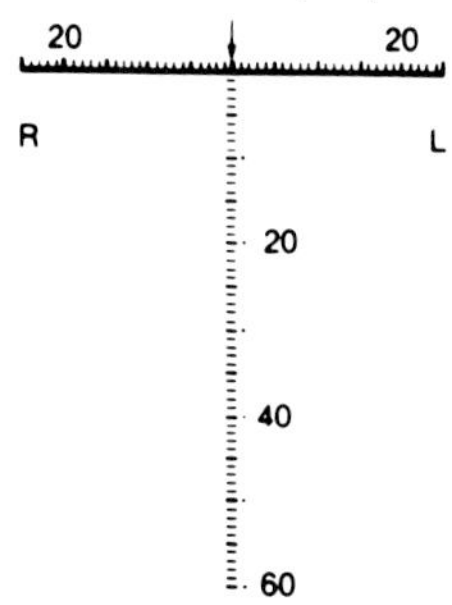

	ACTIVE movement	PAIN R	PAIN L	PASSIVE movement comp. to ACTIVE	PAIN R	PAIN L
maximum mouth opening	____ mm			+ =		
laterotrusion R	____ mm			+ =		
laterotrusion L	____ mm			+ =		
protrusion deviation to:	R L					
retrusion:						

locking	R	L
clicking	R	L
crepitation	R	L

2

type of "endfeel": ____________________

lip, cheek, tongue, palate: ____________________

joint and muscle conditions:

joint tests		R	L	
asymmetrical movements				
limitation of movements				
"joint play" (+ or −)	P			P
lateral tenderness				
posterior tenderness				

joint/muscle dynamic pain R	joint/muscle dynamic pain L		muscle static pain R	muscle static pain L
		opening		
		closing		
		laterotrusion R		
		laterotrusion L		
		protrusion		

muscles tender to palpation: ____________________

movements of the cervical spine:

flexion (45°-55°)	°	P
extension (70°)	°	P

rotation (80°-85°)	R	°	P
	L	°	P
lateroflexion (45°)	R	°	P
	L	°	P

3

Protocol for functional examination of the stomatognathic system by the dentist as described by Hansson et al (1985).

Clinical Observations

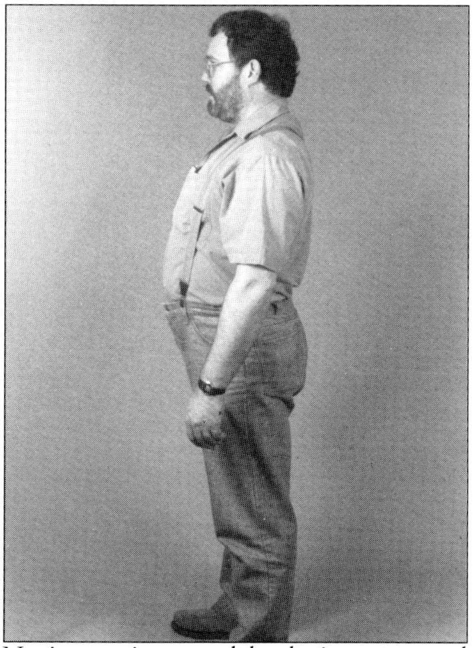

Notice an increased lordotic curve and shoulder retraction.

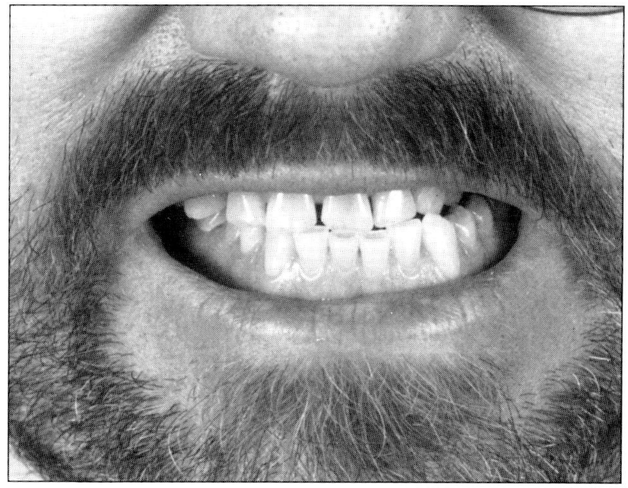

Notice a forward position of the mandible (abused protrusion) and an unequally worn tooth pattern.

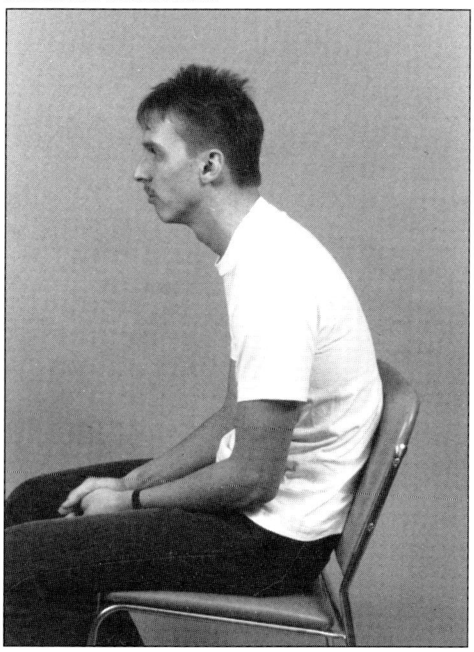

Notice a forward head position in sitting and an increased lower thoracic curve with an absent lordotic curve.

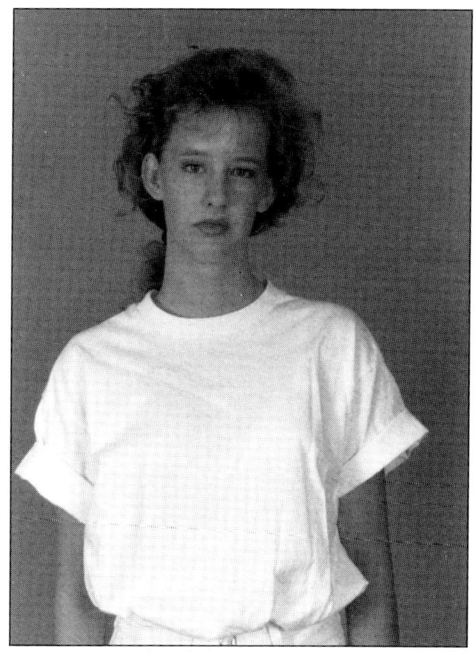

Notice a tilted head position in the frontal plane and an elevated left shoulder.

Clinical Observations

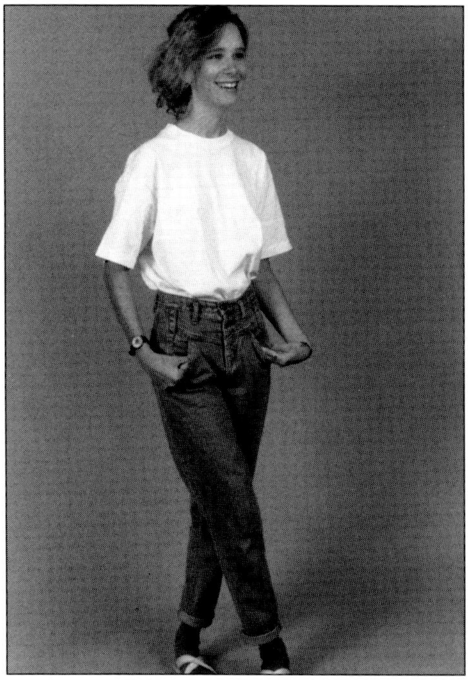

Notice the extreme border positions of the joints at rest (signs of hypermobility). Notice the forward head with a forward mandibular position. Notice rounded shoulders and the marked wrist flexion.

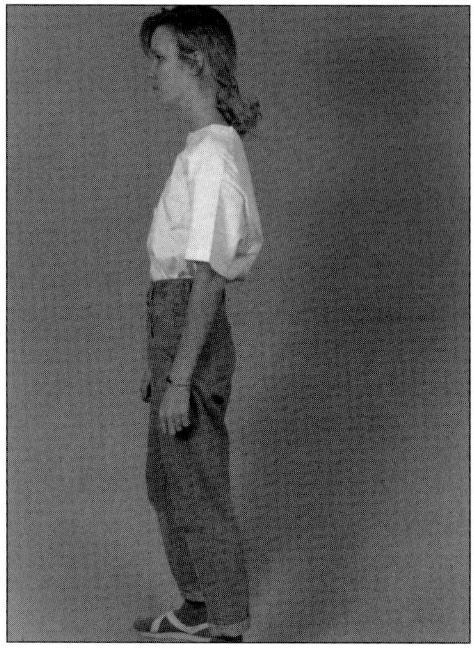

Notice the forward head position and the lack of muscular stabilization in posture.

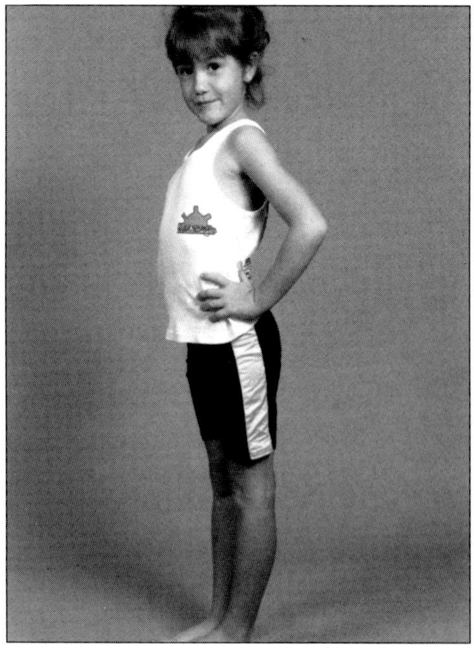

Notice the increased lumbar lordosis and the genu recurvatum.

Clinical Observations

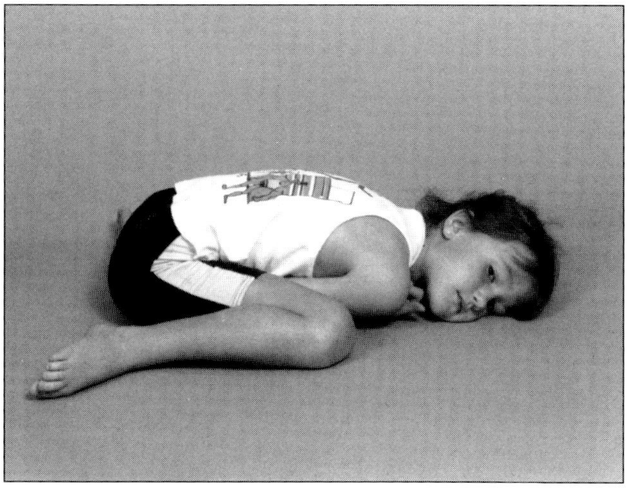

Notice the extreme border positions of the joints at rest.

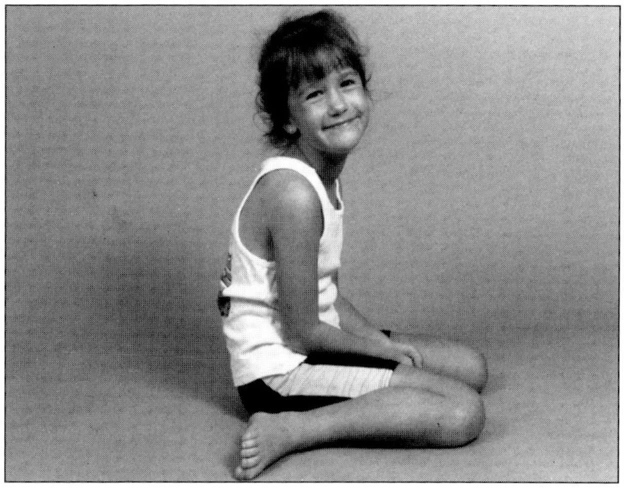

Notice the extreme border positions of the joints in sitting and the obvious lack of muscular stabilization in sitting posture.

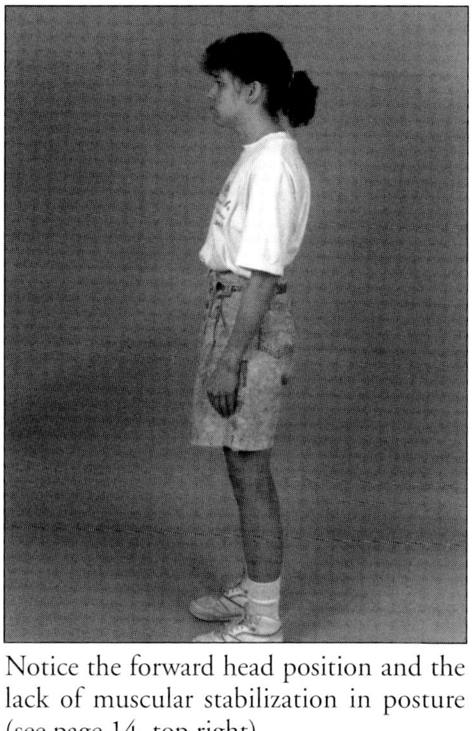

Notice the forward head position and the lack of muscular stabilization in posture (see page 14, top right).

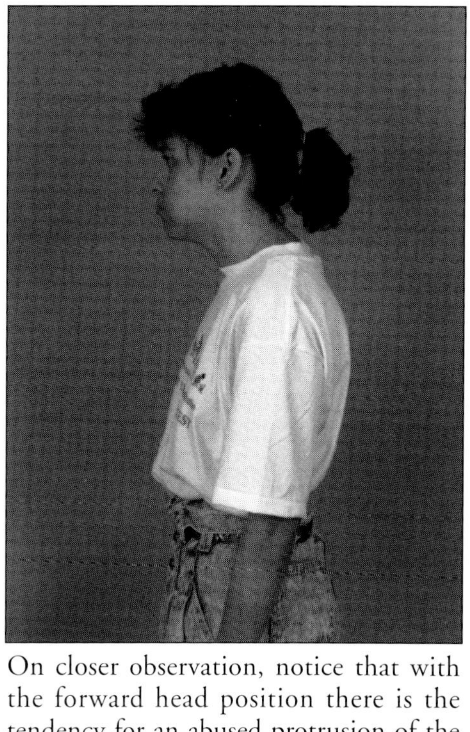

On closer observation, notice that with the forward head position there is the tendency for an abused protrusion of the mandible (closer view of previous figure).

Protocol

2

To assist and organize the multiple areas needed for a complete evaluation of CMD, the following examination protocol is suggested. The protocol makes the examination concise. It is easy to use and assesses what needs to be improved in the condition of the patient. Initially the patient completes his or her self-assessment to familiarize the examiner with the patient's perception of his or her symptoms and diagnosis (see page 19). It also provides a treatment history, as many patients have been seen by multiple professionals. This guides the examiner-therapist in creating the treatment plan and helps avoid duplicating treatment; at the same time, it builds the patient's self-consciousness and growing responsibility for participation regarding his or her CMD. It is also a tool that assists the therapist in the final phase of the treatment as he or she reassesses the progress. As patients begin to progress, they forget at times how severe their pain and decreased function were initially.

In the self-assessment, the patients rate their own pain and explain their pain and how it affects them in their daily activities.

During the cervical evaluation (see page 20), posture, strength, and active cervical range of motion are evaluated (see pages 21 through 31). If there is a limitation of active movement or if there is pain, the movements are then tested passively. It is also necessary to examine upper extremity range of motion because many patients have tight pectoral muscles, which is a limitation for maintaining posture. In addition, upper extremity strength is also important to test. Many patients clench their teeth when making a physical effort in order to get all the "assistance" they can.

At the palpation of the cervical area and shoulder girdle, the following items are emphasized and compared: hypertrophy, hypotrophy, hypersensitivity, hyposensitivity. The patient's right and left sides are always compared to establish the norm and muscle balance. Not until this information is gathered will it be possible to understand why a patient is unable to hold a functioning posture.

In the evaluation of the masticatory system, only the most obvious features are stressed: tenderness, how the movements of the mouth are performed, and posture-habits of the mandible during the examination (see pages 32 through 37).

In the examination of the joint noises there are basically two different noises to distinguish: clicking and crepitation. Clicking sounds indicate local irregularities of the articulating components with or without internal derangement of an anteriorly displaced TMJ disc. A clinical way of identifying the most likely cause for the sound is to determine when and where the clicking sound occurs during the mandibular movements of opening and closing. If the sound occurs only on opening, only on closing, or on opening and on closing in the same mandibular position, it is due to irregularities of the articulating components. If the sound occurs on opening and on closing and in different mandibular positions, it is caused by a displaced disc that is in the wrong relationship with its condyle.

Crepitation is a longer sound and of a cracking nature. Its existence is explained by the presence of deteriorated articulating surfaces, most often a disc perforation in combination with some other degenerative changes in the temporal component and condyle. Crepitation is mostly observed among elderly persons. However, crepitation can also be heard in younger joints, where it is more likely caused by inflammatory changes of the synovial membrane.

Joint noises alone (ie, without any pain or other signs of a disorder) are not an indication for treatment. These noises can be checked over a longer period of time and most often they remain asymptomatic.

Not until the mandibular measurements are completed (see page 38) is the overall joint mobility determined as hypomobile, normal, or hypermobile. As an average, the laterotrusive movements of the mandible are approximately one fourth the maximum mouth opening (Agerberg 1974).

Joint play is performed as a traction and as a translation of the condyle-disc complex from the temporal component; pain is observed. Traction involves the joint components as well as the vertical portions of the masticatory muscles in the surrounding area of the joint capsule. Translation involves the articulating components and the horizontal portions of the masticatory muscles that direct the function of the TMJ (see page 39). (Note: translation can provide information about irregularities and lesions of the articulating components of the joint.)

A final step in the manipulation of the joint components is a slightly retrusive guidance of the mandible from the rest position without tooth contacts. It should be noted if pain is elicited in the right or left TMJ region (see page 40).

By identifying the dysfunction, the preliminary diagnosis (ie, the reason for physical therapy) is confirmed or rejected (see page 41). At this time a treatment plan is designed that sets measurable short-term and long-term goals. Within a specified time of treatment the goals must be achieved. Should the predicted results not be attained, the condition requires reevaluation by the treatment team.

Because the patient has already been thoroughly examined by the dentist, there is no reason for the physical therapist to give priority to the dentition. If occlusal factors have been found to play a major role in the development of the CMD, generally an artificial occlusion in the form of a splint fakes the occlusion and does not require any further attention other than that given regularly by the dentist (see page 42).

St. Joseph's Hospital
and Medical Center
Outpatient Physical Therapy

PATIENT'S SELF ASSESSMENT

NAME: ________________________ PATIENT NUMBER ____________

AGE: ______ TODAY'S DATE ____________ YOUR DIAGNOSIS ______________

REFERRING DOCTOR/DENTIST ________________ OCCUPATION: ____________

Briefly describe your present problem in your own words (e.g., pain, numbness, weakness, etc.):

When did your problem begin and how did your problem start? ______________

If this is an on-going problem, when did it worsen? ______________

What treatment have you had so far (or are you presently receiving)? ______________

PAIN: ☐ Constant ☐ Intermittent (comes and goes)

Aggravated/worsened by: ______________

Relieved by: ______________

Location: Please use the pain drawing and codes to show where your pain is.

= sharp

= shooting

= tightness/dull pain

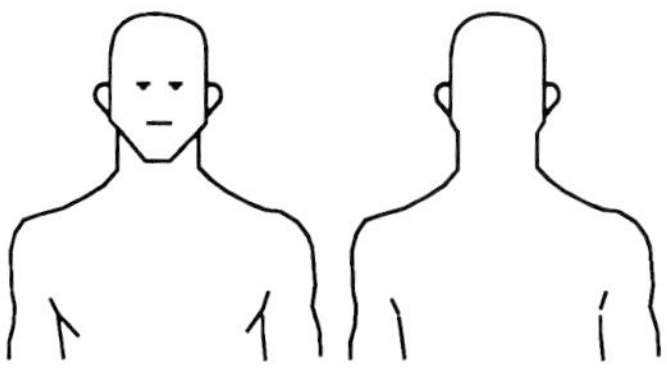

Intensity: Please rate your pain on the following scale (0 = no pain, 10 = worst imaginable pain):

0 1 2 3 4 5 6 7 8 9 10

FUNCTION: Please list any activities that you are now unable to do because of your present problem:

Feel free to give any other information related to your problem: ______________

Do you have any medical problems? ______________

Are you under a doctor's care for any problem other than what we are seeing you for?

OPD-2076

Page 1 in the physical therapy examination protocol: self-assessment.

CERVICAL EVALUATION

Patient Name ____________________

Patient Number ____________________

POSTURE:

Forward head: ____________________ Rounded shoulders: ____________________

Kyphotic: ____________________ Increased lordotic curve: ____________________

ACTIVE CERVICAL RANGE OF MOTION:

Flexion (45° - 55°)	______	P	Extension (70°)		______	P
Rotation (80° - 85°)	R ______	P	Lateroflexion (45°)	R	______	P
	L ______	P		L	______	P

Comments: ____

____

PASSIVE CERVICAL MOBILITY: ____________________

ACTIVE UPPER EXTREMITY RANGE OF MOTION:

Shoulder Flexion (160° - 180°)	R ______	P	Shoulder Abduction (120°)	R ______	P
	L ______	P		L ______	P

Comments: ____

____

RESISTED CERVICAL MOTIONS:

Flexion	______	P	Extension	______	P
Rotation	R ______	P	Lateroflexion	R ______	P
	L ______	P		L ______	P

KEY
1 = Trace
2 = Poor
3 = Fair
4 = Good
5 = Normal

UPPER EXTREMITY STRENGTH:

Shoulder Flexion	R ______	P	Shoulder Abduction	R ______	P
	L ______	P		L ______	P
Scapular Muscles	R ______	P			
	L ______	P			

Number of shoulder shrugs: ______

Comments: ____

____

TENDERNESS TO PALPATION:

Sternocleidomastoid	R ______	L ______	Trapezius	R ______	L ______
Scaleni	R ______	L ______	Suboccipitals	R ______	L ______
Levator Scapula	R ______	L ______	Rhomboids	R ______	L ______

-2-

Page 2 in the physical therapy examination protocol: cervical evaluation.

Posture Evaluation

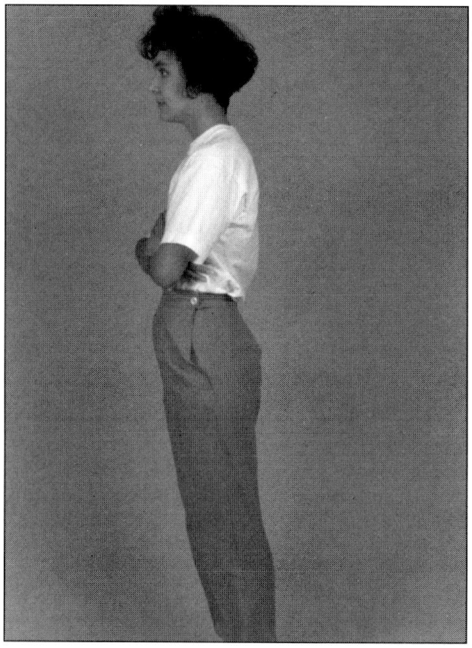

Forward head position and an increased lordotic curve.

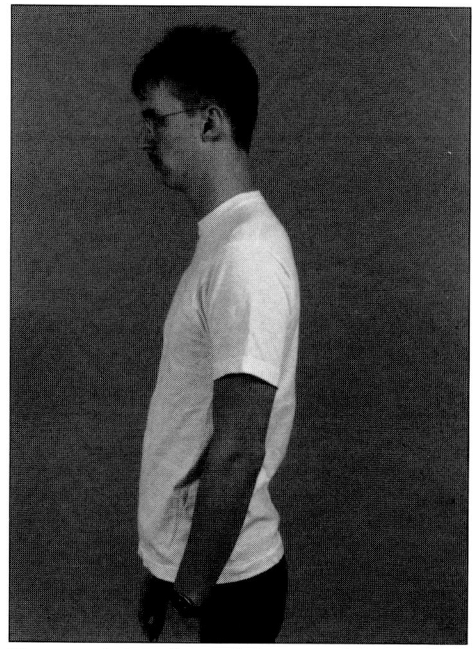

Forward head position and rounded shoulders. Lack of muscular stabilization.

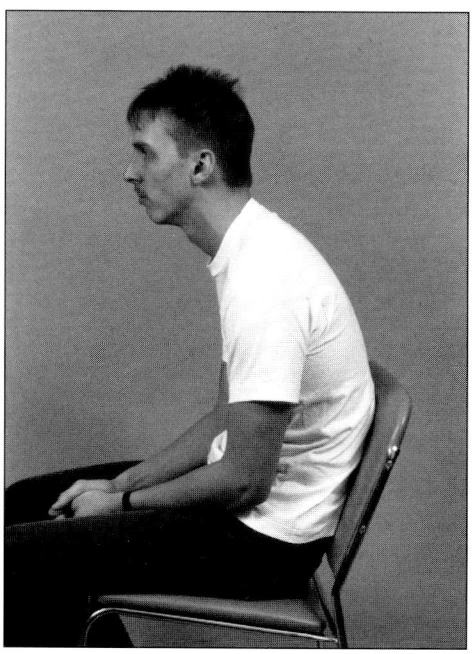

Forward head position and rounded shoulders. Absence of lordotic curve. Notice the difference between the sitting and standing postures (see figure at top right).

Active Cervical Range of Motion

Measurements with the Aid of a Goniometer

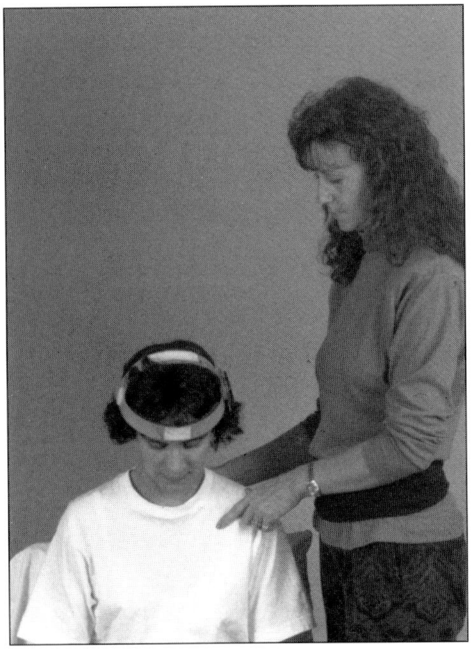

Flexion.

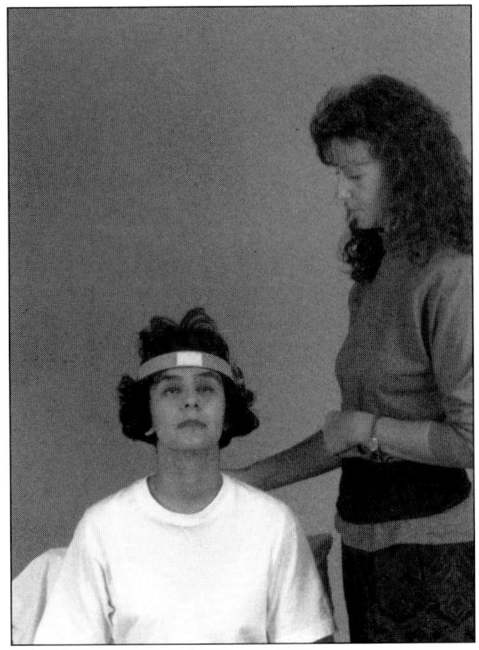

Extension.

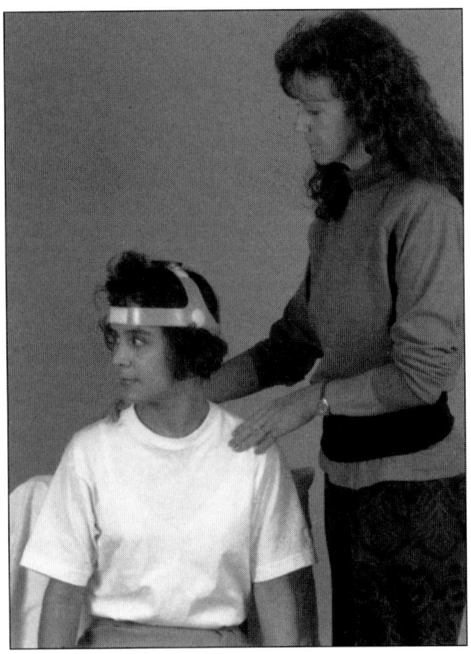

Rotation to the right.

Active Cervical Range of Motion

Measurements with the Aid of a Goniometer

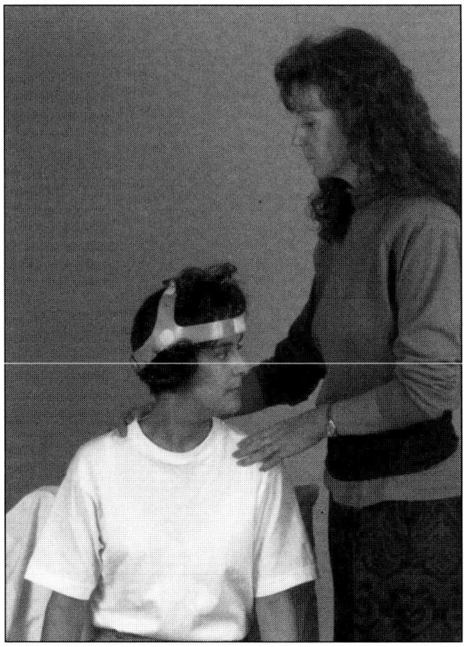

Rotation to the left.

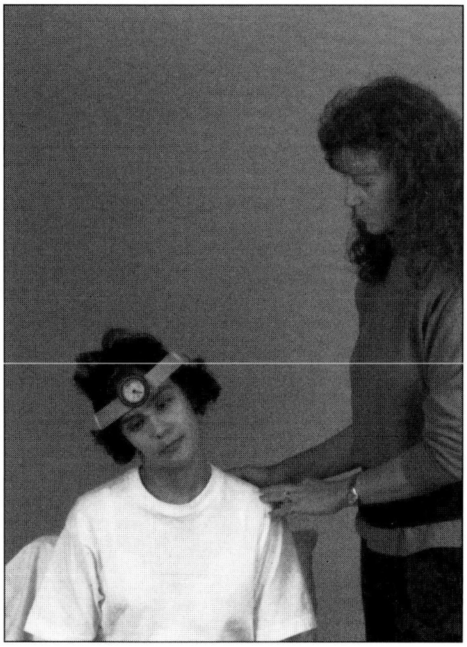

Lateroflexion right.

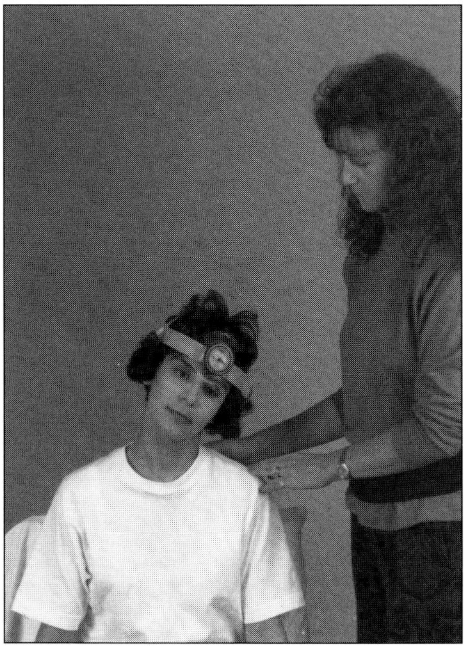

Lateroflexion left.

Passive Cervical Range of Motion

Evaluation

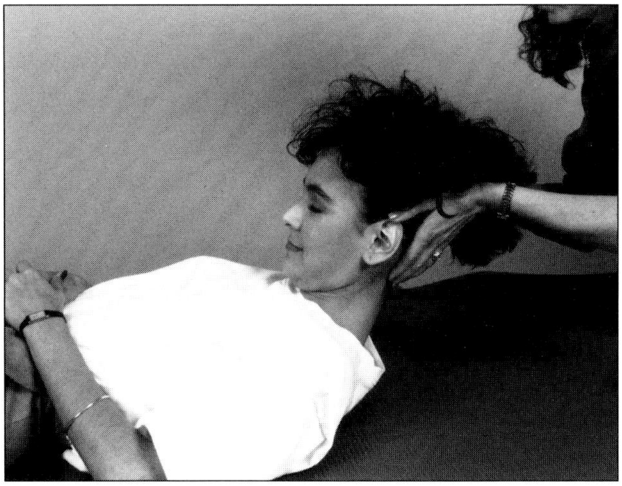

Flexion. Note the quality of resistance (end feel) and locate limitations.

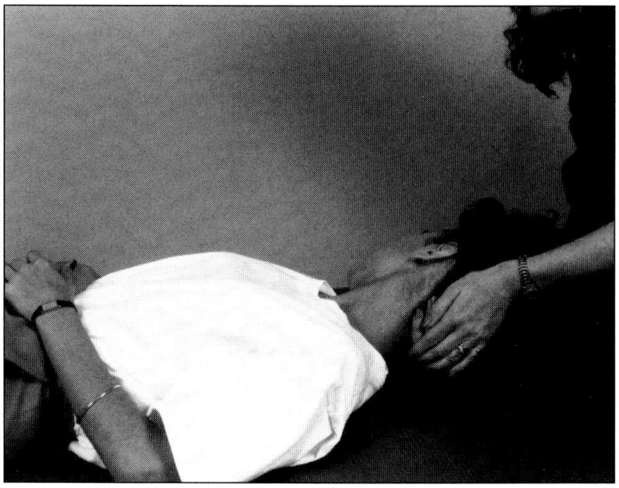

Rotation to the right. Note the quality of resistance (end feel) and locate limitations.

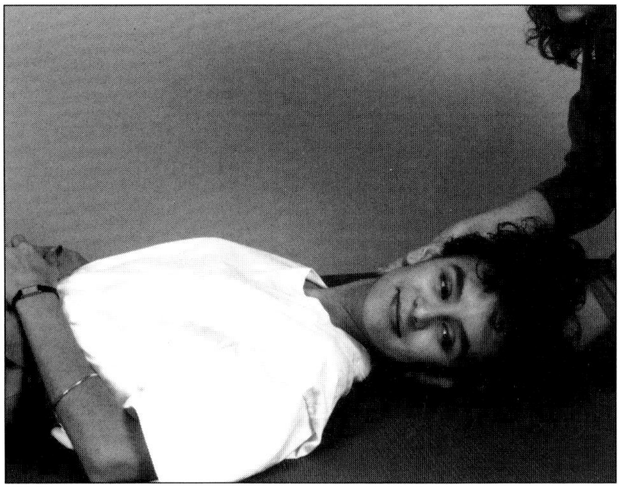

Rotation to the left. Note the quality of resistance (end feel) and locate limitations.

Passive Cervical Range of Motion

Evaluation

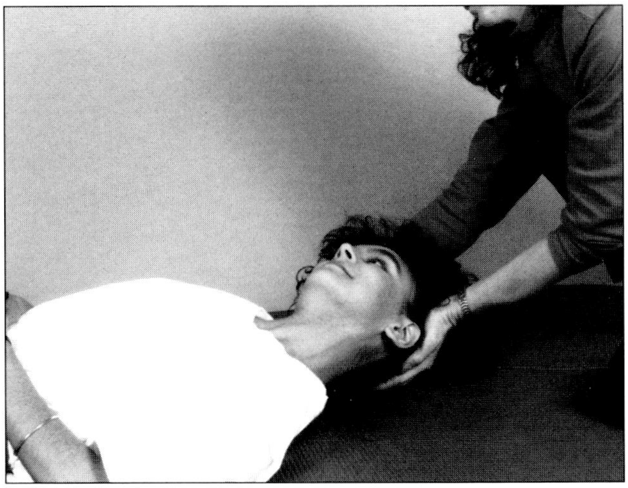

Lateroflexion right. Note the quality of resistance (end feel) and locate limitations.

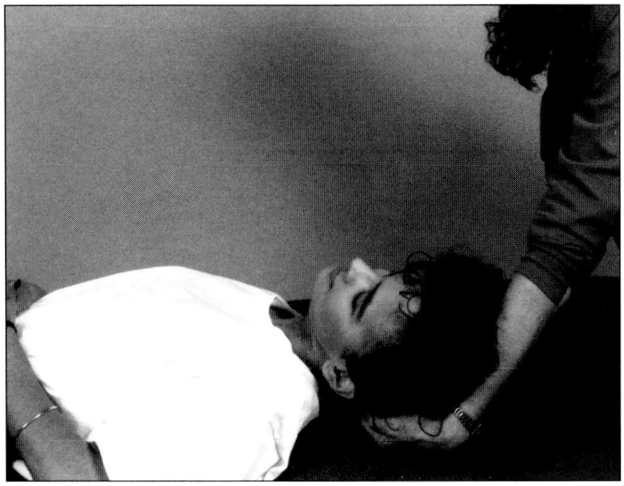

Lateroflexion left. Note the quality of resistance (end feel) and locate limitations.

Active Upper-Extremity Range of Motion

Measurements

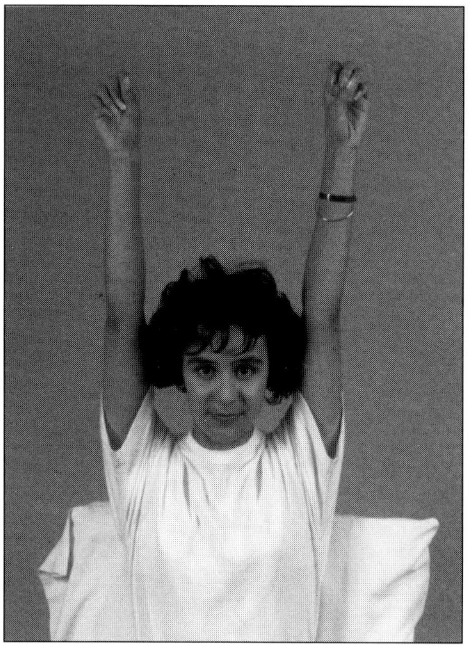

Shoulder flexion. Note limitations and their effects on posture.

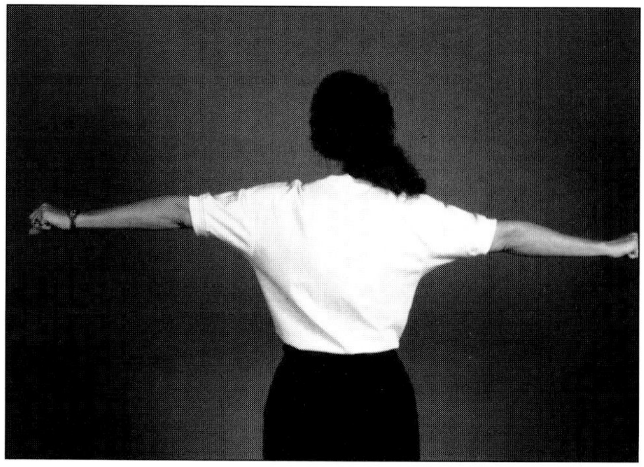

Shoulder abduction. Note limitations and their effects on posture.

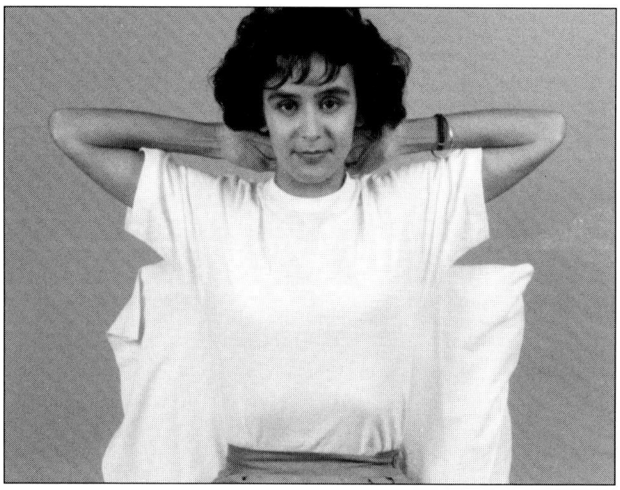

Shoulder abduction with external rotation. Note limitations and their effects on posture.

Resisted Cervical Motions

Evaluation

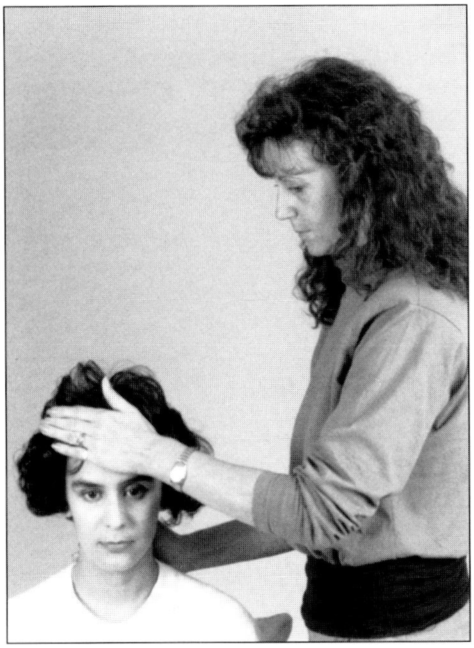

Flexion. Note strength and the response to the applied resistance (pain and its location).

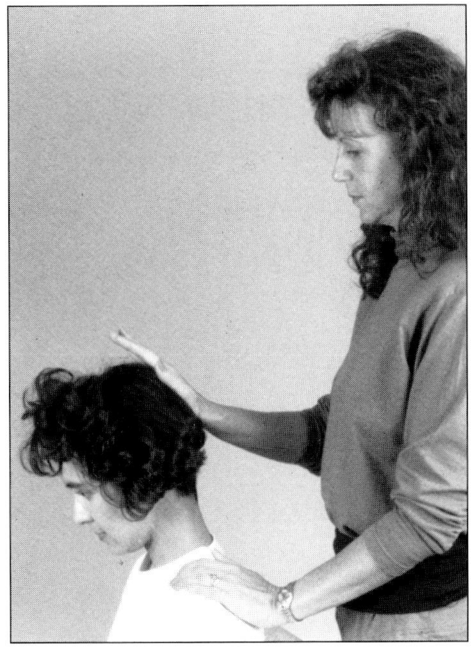

Extension. Note strength and the response to the applied resistance (pain and its location).

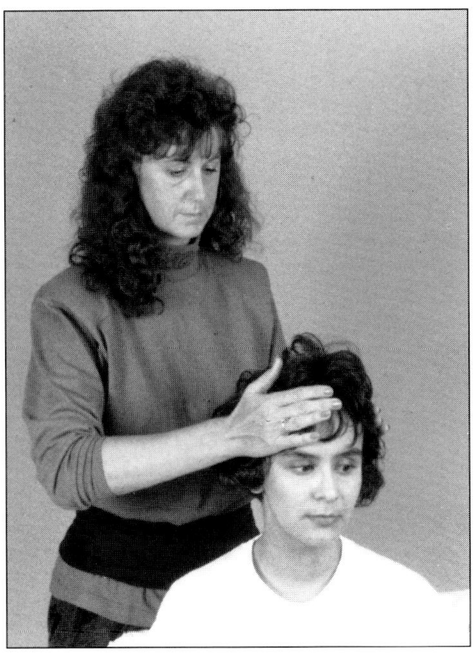

Rotation to the right. Note strength and the response to the applied resistance (pain and its location).

Resisted Cervical Motions

Evaluation

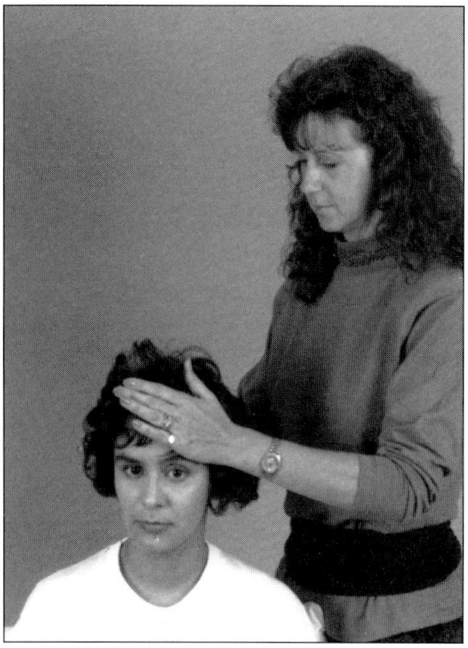

Rotation to the left. Note strength and the response to the applied resistance (pain and its location).

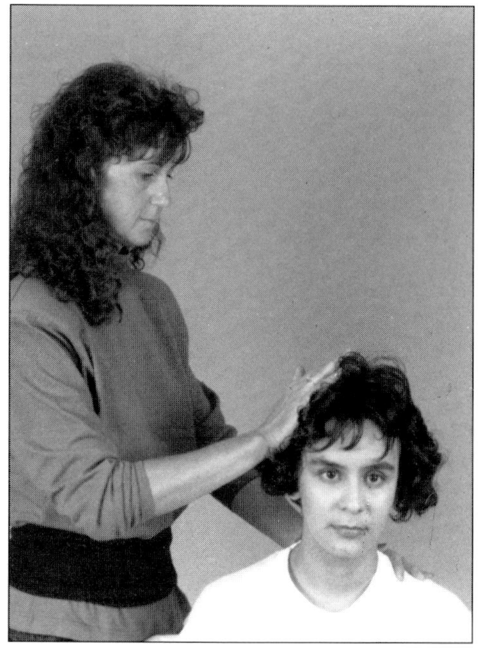

Lateroflexion right. Note strength and the response to the applied resistance (pain and its location).

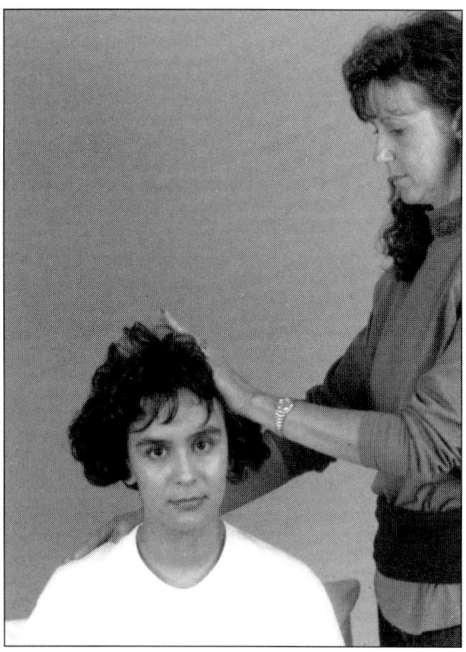

Lateroflexion left. Note strength and the response to the applied resistance (pain and its location).

Upper Extremity Strength

Evaluation

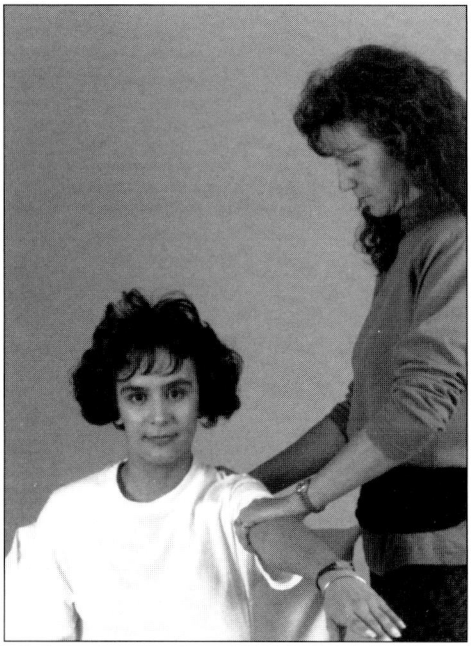

Shoulder flexion. Note strength and the response to the applied resistance (pain and its location).

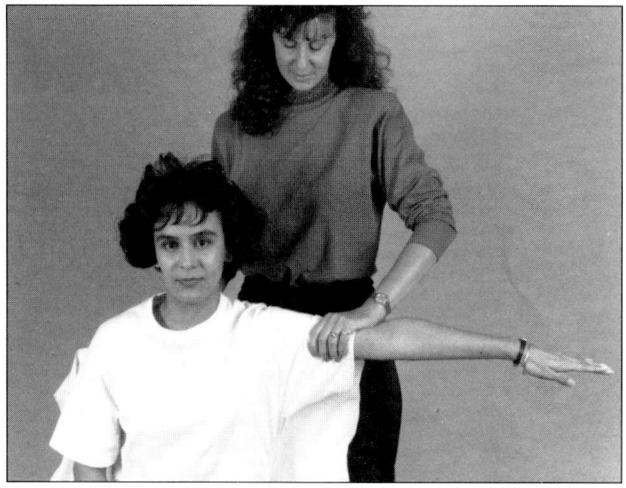

Shoulder abduction. Note strength and the response to the applied resistance (pain and its location).

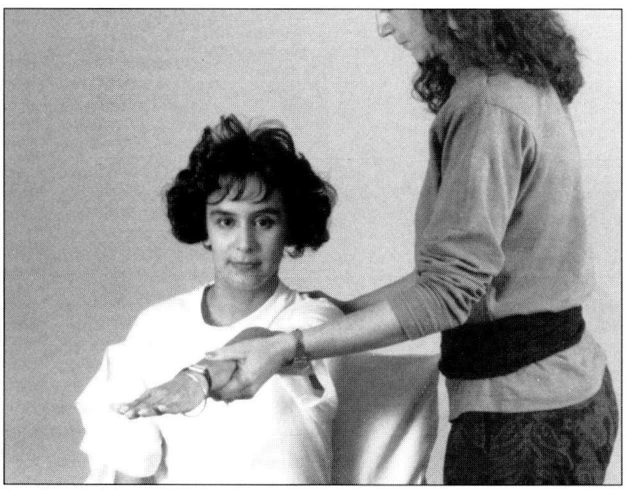

Horizontal abduction. Note strength and the response to the applied resistance (pain and its location).

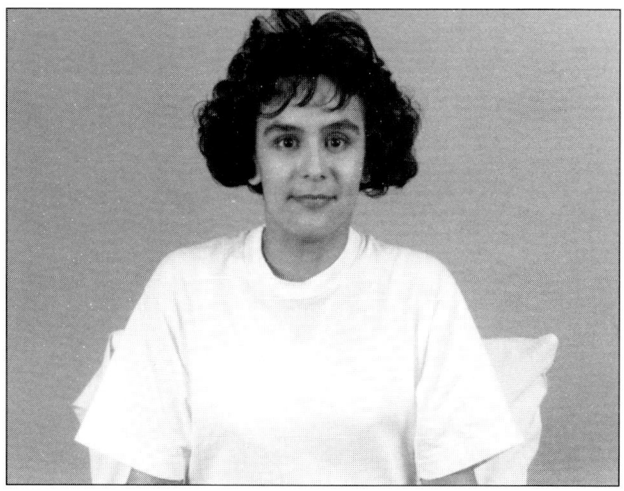

Shoulder elevation–shrug. Note strength and the response to the resistance when applied (pain and its location).

Palpation of the Upper Quarter

Patient's Response

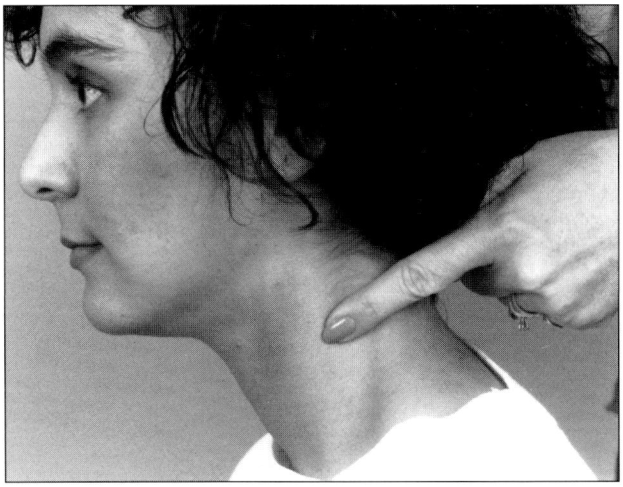

Musculus sternocleidomastoideus.

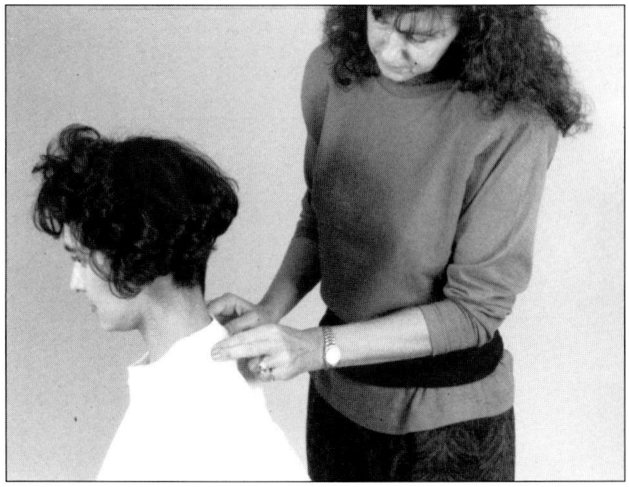

Musculus trapezius.

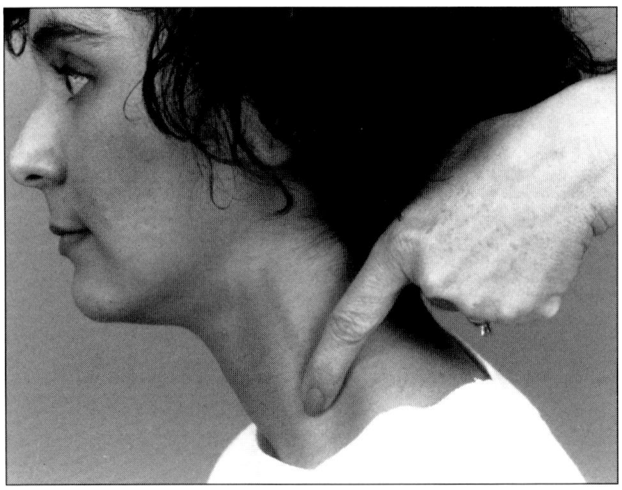

Musculi scaleni.

Palpation of the Upper Quarter

Patient's Response

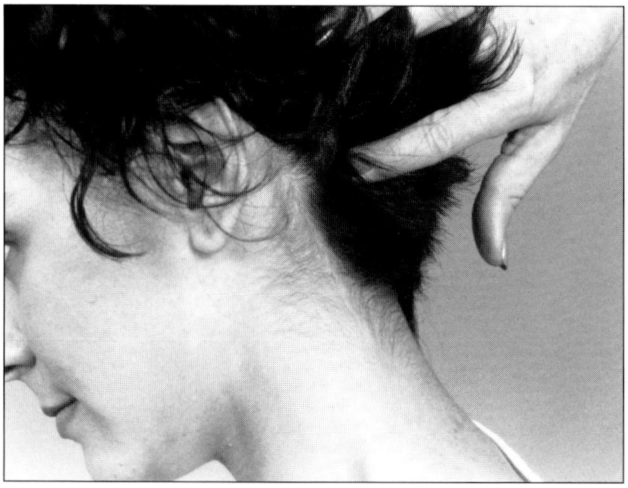

Musculus suboccipitalis.

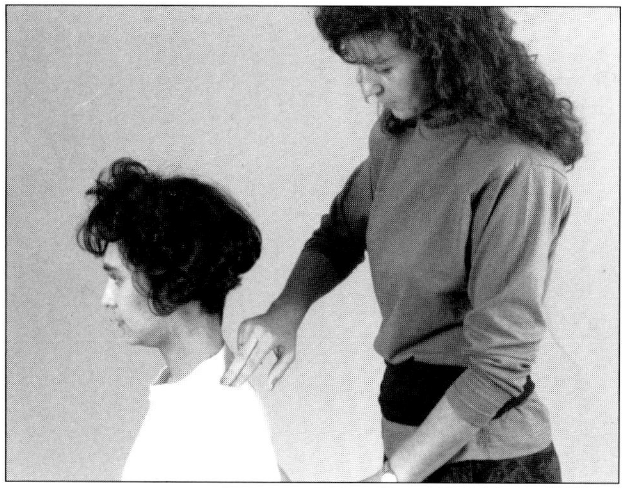

Musculus levator scapulae.

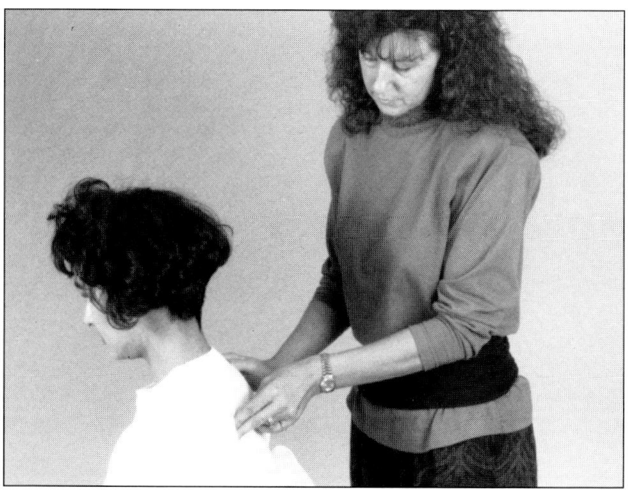

Musculus rhomboideus.

TMJ EVALUATION

Patient Name ____________________

Patient Number ____________________

TENDERNESS TO PALPATION:

Masseter	R ________	L ________
Temporalis	R ________	L ________
Medial Pterygoid	R ________	L ________
TMJ Lateral Pole	R ________	L ________

Comments: ____

____

MECHANICS:

Maximum opening: ________ mm [P]

Deviation:	☐ Yes	☐ No	Right	P	Left	P
Deflection:	☐ Yes	☐ No	Right	P	Left	P
Joint Noises:	☐ Yes	☐ No	Right	P	Left	P

Describe: ________________________________

Where: ________________________________

Protrusion:	________ mm	P
Left laterotrusion:	________ mm	P
Right laterotrusion:	________ mm	P

Mouth opening/closing deviation (mm)

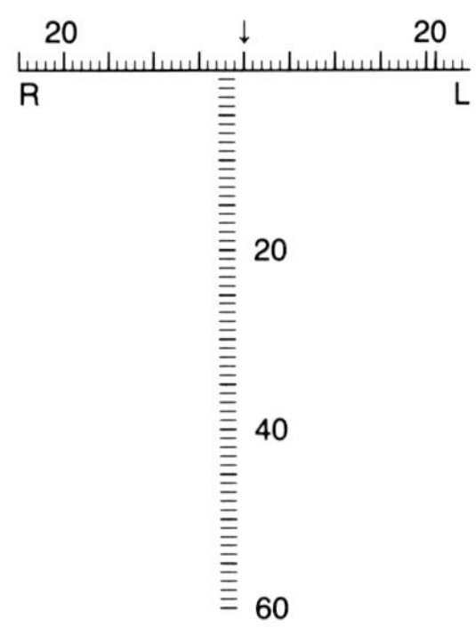

OVERALL JOINT MOBILITY:

1 = hypomobile 2 = normal 3 = hypermobile

JOINT PLAY:

Distraction:	Right	P	Left	P
Translation:	Right	P	Left	P

Retrusive overpressure: Right ________ [P] Left ________ [P]

OTHER: ____

____

____

____

____

-3-

Page 3 in the physical therapy examination protocol: TMJ evaluation.

Palpation of the Masticatory Muscles

Patient's Response

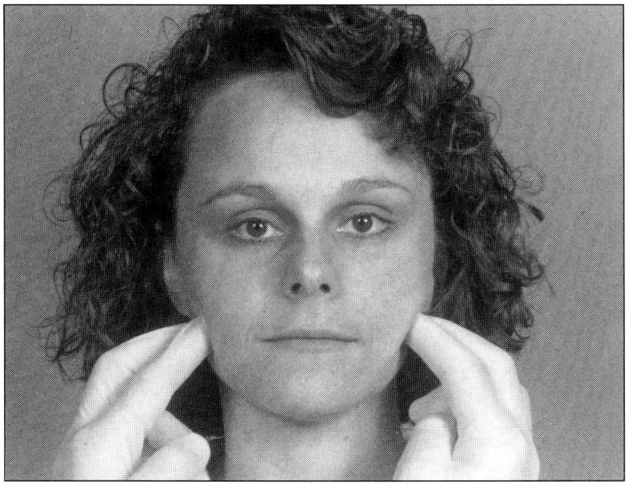

Bilateral palpation denotes the difference in pain response between the two sides. Musculus masseter.

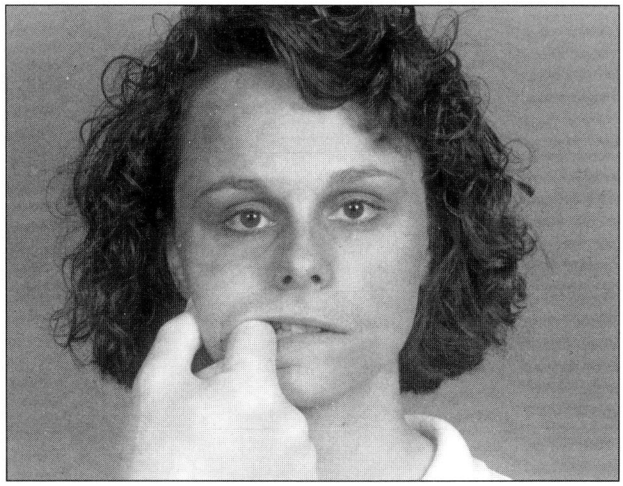

Unilateral palpation denotes the difference in pain response within the muscle. Musculus masseter.

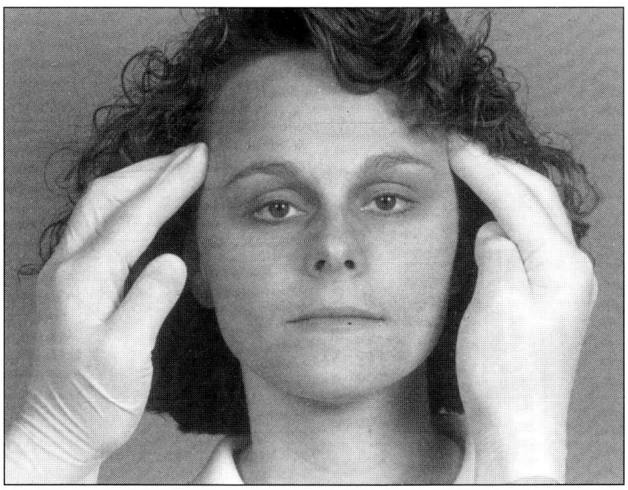

Bilateral palpation denotes the difference in pain response between the two sides. Musculus temporalis.

Palpation of the Masticatory Muscles

Patient's Response

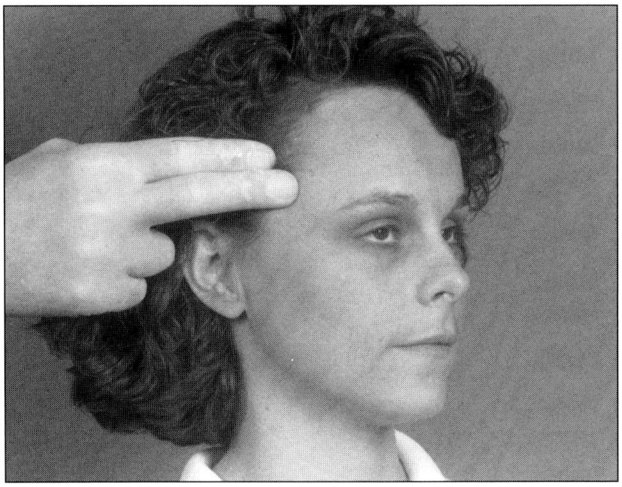

Vertical portion of the temporal muscle (musculus temporalis).

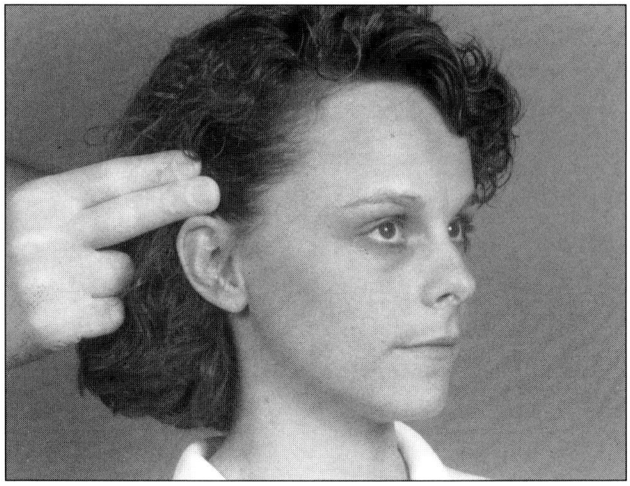

Horizontal portion of the temporal muscle (musculus temporalis).

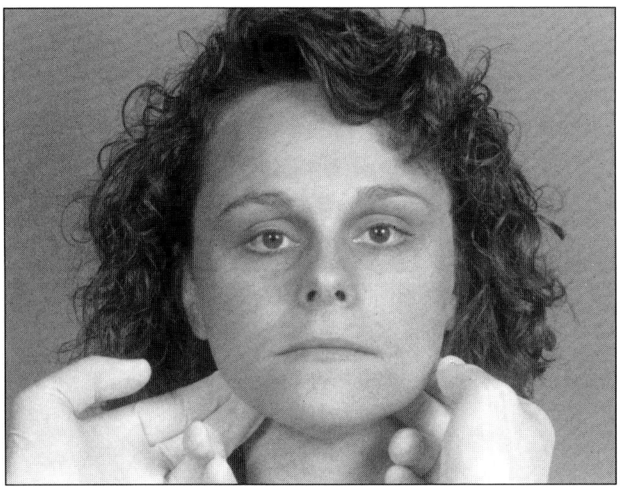

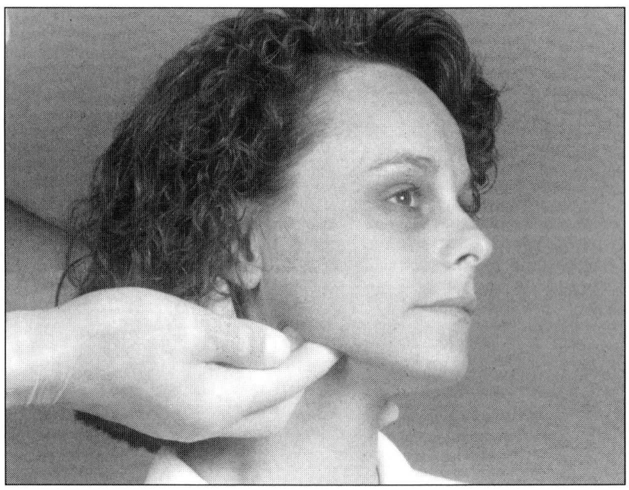

Bilateral palpation denotes the difference in pain response between the two sides. Musculus pterygoideus medialis.

Palpation of the Lateral Pole of the TMJ

Patient's Response

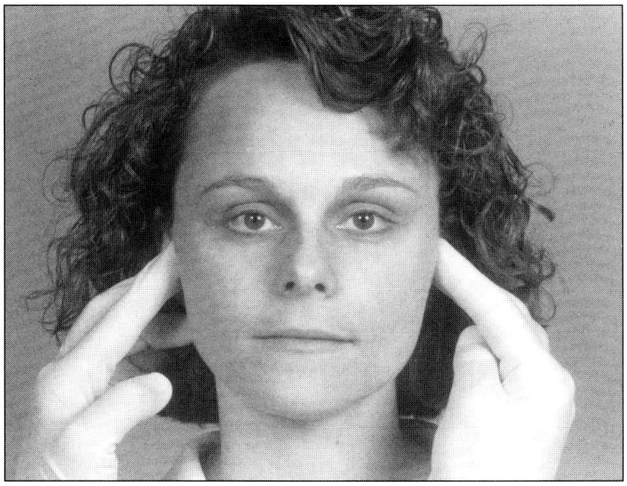

Bilateral palpation denotes the difference in pain response between the two TMJs. Mandible in rest position.

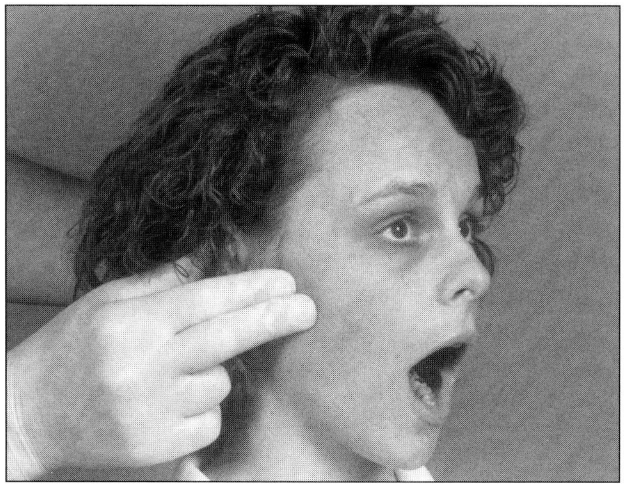

During mouth opening.

Mechanics

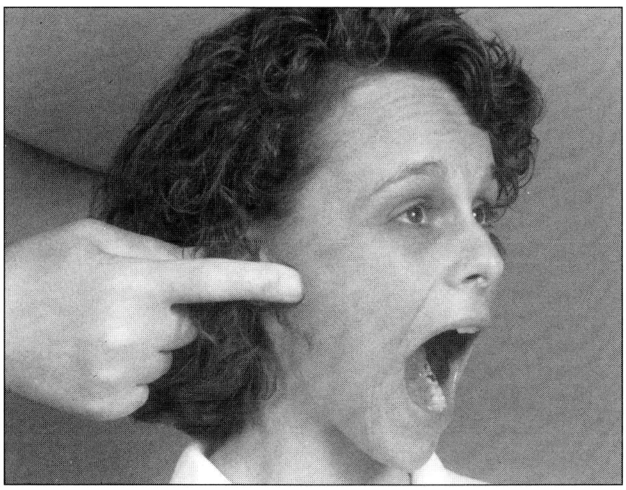

Notice the movement of the TMJ condylar head during mouth opening.

Mandibular Movements

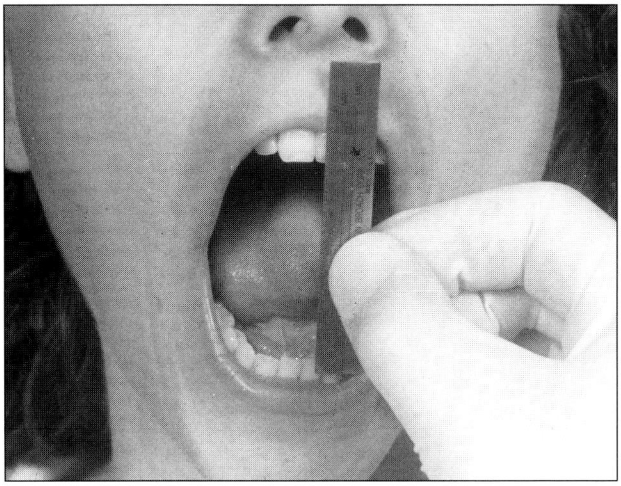

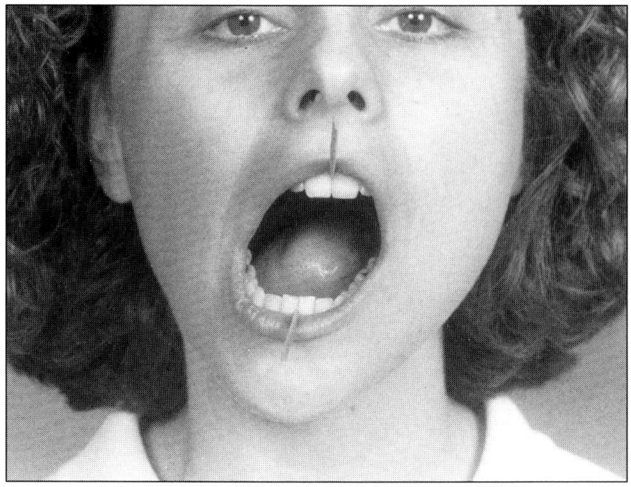

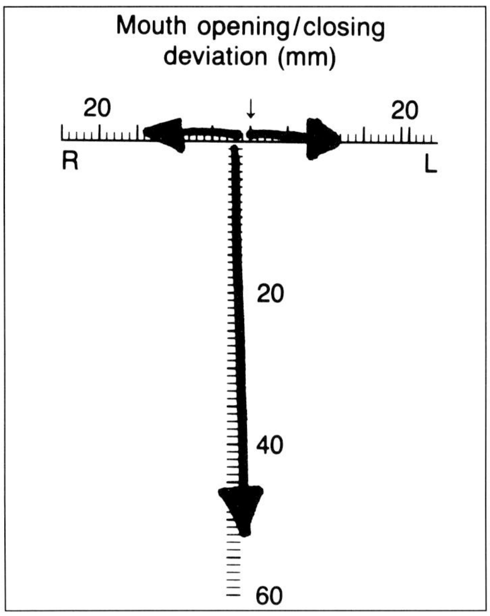

Active maximum mouth opening is measured as the distance between the incisal edges of the maxillary and mandibular central anterior teeth, expressed in millimeters. Average values of maximum mouth opening vary between 45 and 55 mm. Notice when the vertical overbite is extensive (ie, when half of the buccal surfaces of the mandibular teeth are covered by the maxillary teeth or more in maximum occlusion). Include this observation in your evaluation of the maximum mouth opening. Note pain and its location.

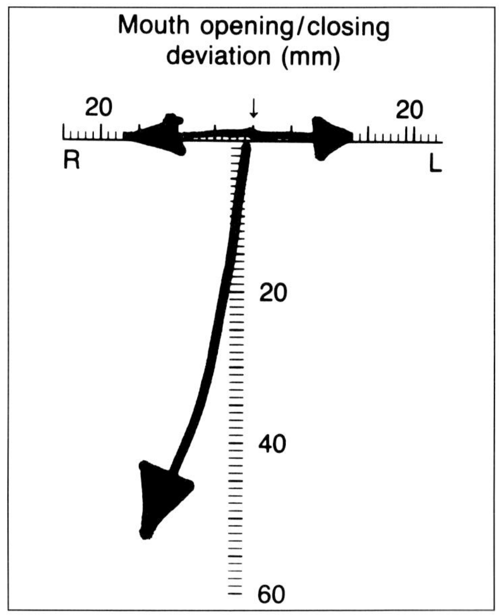

Deviation of the mandible to the right on maximum mouth opening. Note the deviation of the chin point to the right.

Mandibular Movements

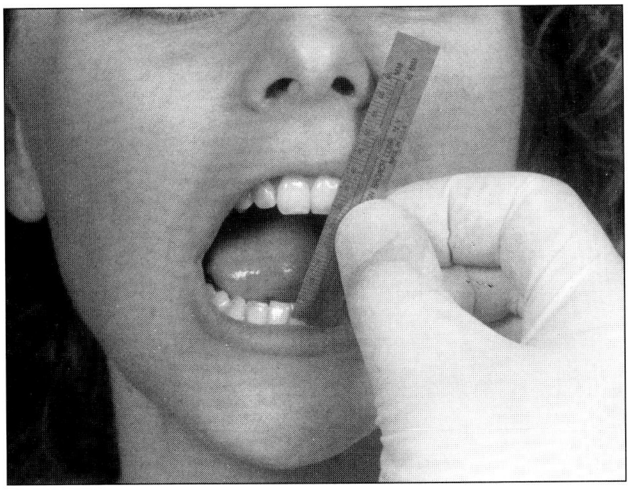

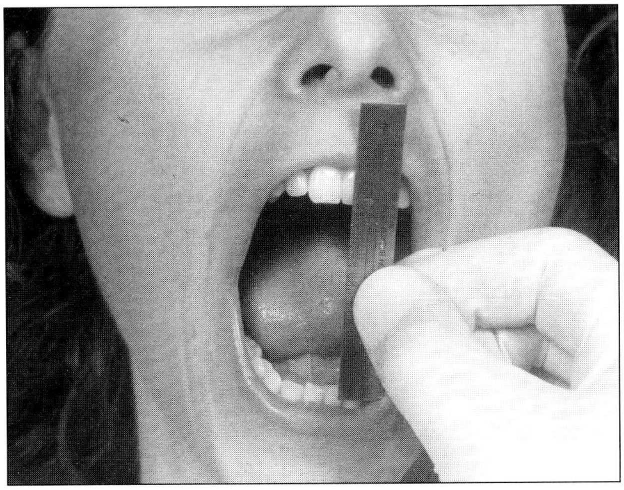

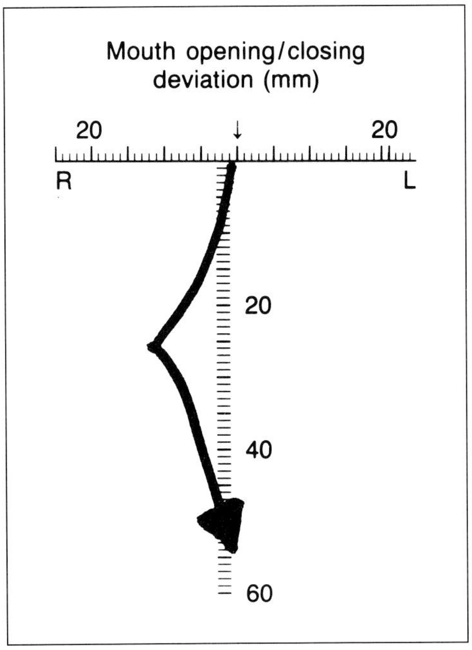

Deflection of the mandible to the right during mouth opening. Note the symmetrical end position of the chin at maximum mouth opening.

Mandibular Movements

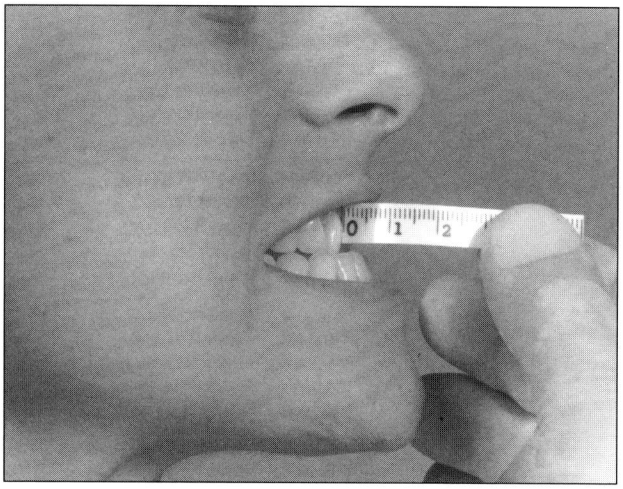

Protrusion.

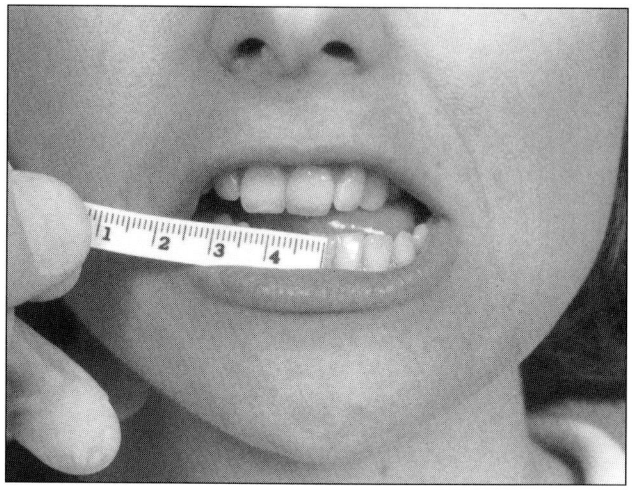

Laterotrusion to the left.

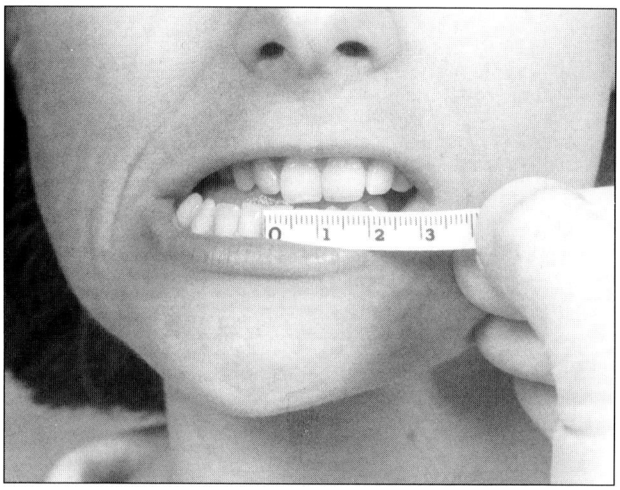

Laterotrusion to the right. As an average, the laterotrusive movements of the mandible are approximately one fourth the maximum mouth opening (Agerberg 1974).

Joint Play

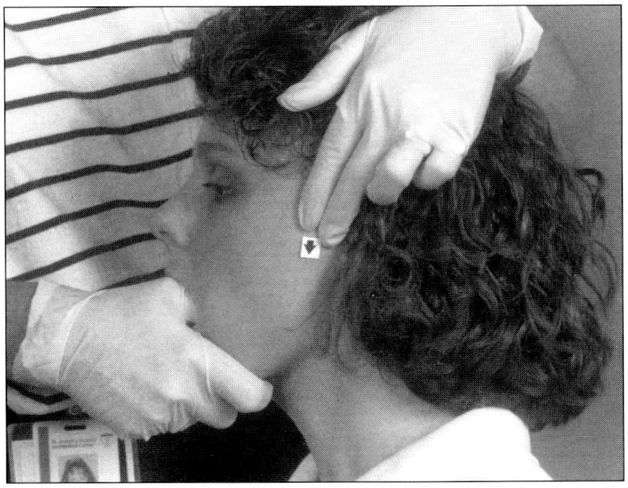

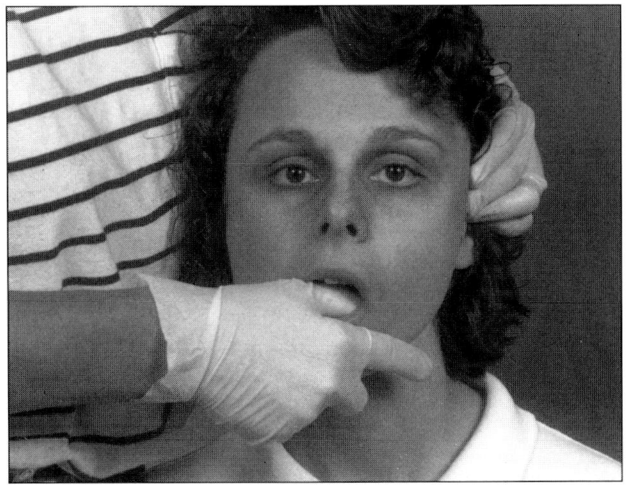

Traction. The head is fixed. The manipulating hand is pushing with its thumb straight downward on the molars of the mandible.

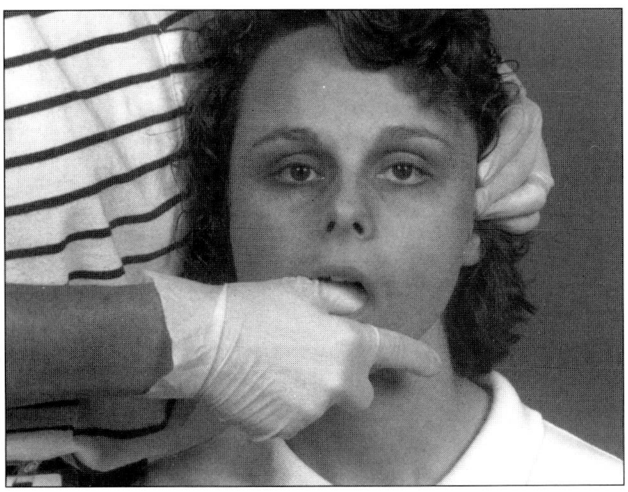

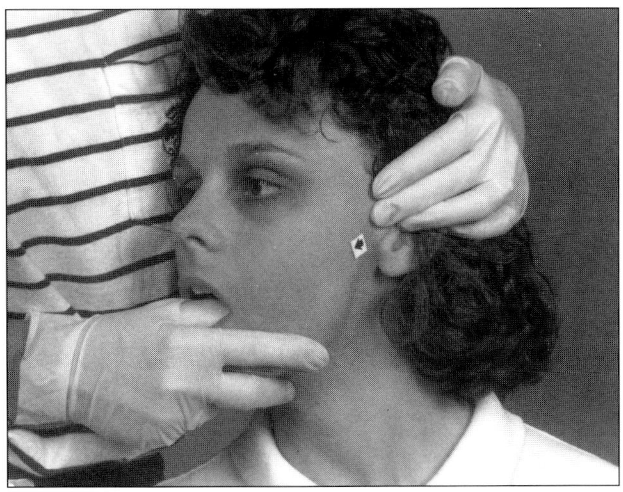

Translation. The head is fixed. The thumb of the manipulating hand is placed on the ipsilateral molars and the index and long fingers are placed exteriorly around the body of the mandible. The manipulating hand is pulling the mandible forward to the contralateral side.

Retrusion of Mandible at Rest

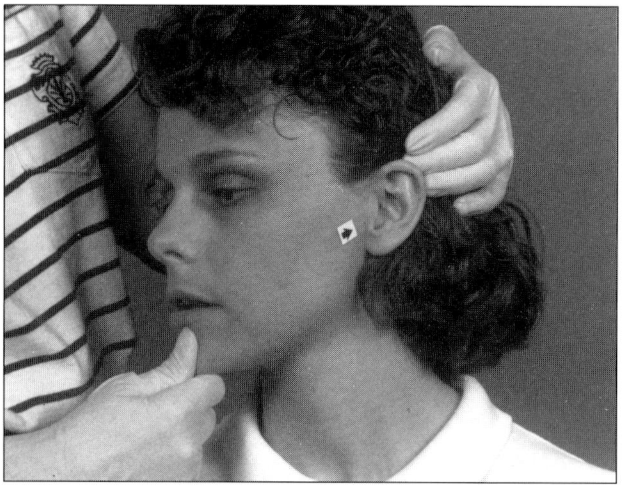

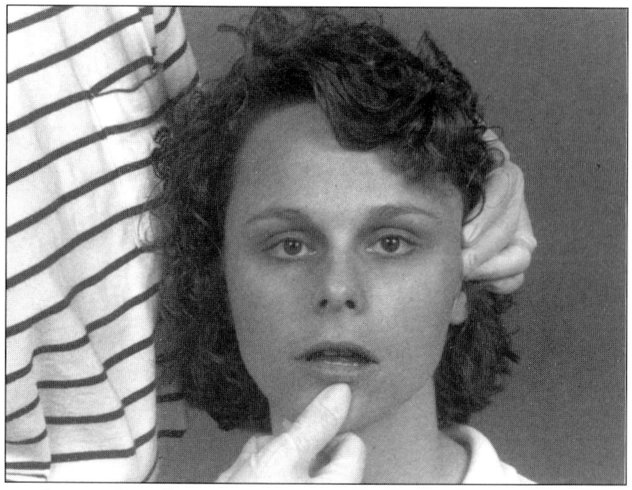

A slight guidance of the manipulating hand may elicit pain in the area of the TMJ. The pain often indicates an ongoing inflammatory process in the soft tissue structures of the disc and capsule.

Changes noted/reported when posture was corrected: ____________________

Clinical impression/assessment: ____________________

Problem List	Short Term Goals	Long Term Goals

Treatment Plan: ____________________

Preliminary diagnosis from the referring doctor: ____________________

SIGNATURE   DATE

-4-

Page 4 in the physical therapy examination protocol: final page.

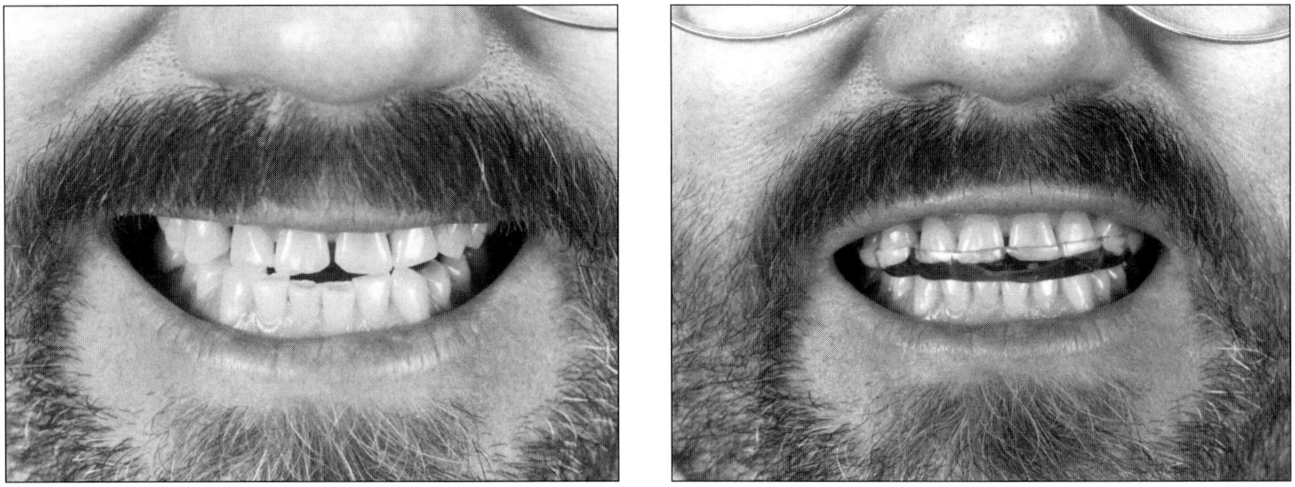

The aim of the splint is to fill empty spaces between the maxillary and mandibular teeth to increase the occlusal stability.

Treatment

3

When the facial pain associated with CMD is determined to be caused by adverse loading of the stomatognathic system, regardless of emotional or morphological reasons, the first attempt in changing the adverse loading must be to remove it. In the clinical situation this is accomplished by PT or a combination of PT and reversible dental treatment in the form of an improved "faked" occlusion through the insertion of an intermaxillary splint (see page 42).

When no major laterally forcing interferences between the retruded contact position (RCP) of the mandible and the intercuspal position (ICP) are present, PT will be the first and only attempt to eliminate the pain.

When an awkward habit has been identified, the initial management is to eliminate the habit, thus optimizing the chances for recovery of the mandibular functions. The change of such habits must not trigger any additional adverse loading of the stomatognathic system via new asymmetrical muscle or joint function.

Although the stomatognathic system is exceptional in its bilateral design, it does not have to be twice as complicated to treat. It may be that several modalities of PT are unnecessary, because the system possesses a potential for recovery as a result of its bilateral design.

The conditions that can be treated successfully are: hypermobility, hypomobility, bruxism, and abused protrusion.

Hypermobility

Definition: Increased laxity of a joint or multiple joints (see page 46).

Have the patient perform all exercises in front of a mirror. The goal is to increase condylar rotation and decrease condyle-disc translation. The patient should work short sessions, 2 to 5 minutes at a time. Following are the instructions for the patient:

1. Limit mouth opening (see page 47).
   a. Put the tip of the tongue far back against your palate. Open and close the mouth with this tongue position maintained. Repeat several times during short sessions every day.
   b. During yawning, limit the mouth opening by positioning the tongue as noted above.
   c. Avoid taking big bites.
2. Work midline (see page 47). Focus the midpoints of the maxillary and mandibular teeth in front of a mirror when opening and closing the mouth. Repeat several times during short sessions every day.
3. Avoid abusive protrusion (see page 48). Reduce forward movements of the mandible. Emphasize the initial rotation of condylar movements.
4. Improve head position in posture (see page 49). Relax the mandibular movements.
5. Resist mandibular movements (see page 50). Apply gentle pressure toward the direction of the movements performed. Keep the amount of movement limited.
6. General strengthening (see pages 51 through 53). Perform active movements. Progress to a low weight strengthening program (1 to 3 pounds).

Hypomobility

Definition: Decreased laxity of a joint or multiple joints (see page 54).

Have the patient sit in correct posture. The goal of the exercises is to increase condylar rotation and to increase condyle-disc translation. Following are the instructions for the patient.

1. Relax the mandible (see page 55). Drop the mandible with the tongue resting superior in the mouth.
2. Stimulate mandibular movements (see pages 55 and 56). Extend your tight movements by manual techniques and self-stretching.
3. Stimulate muscular movements (see pages 56 and 57). Encourage and practice facial expressions.
4. Move the mandible while talking.
5. Keep a daily record of mouth opening.
6. Do general stretching (see pages 57 through 60).

Bruxism

Definition: Teeth grinding or teeth clenching (see pages 61 and 62).

Treatment goals for bruxism are to stop any overloading and to increase mandibular position awareness. Following are the guidelines for the therapist.

1. Show the facets of teeth (improper dental wear) to the patient (see page 63).
2. Help the patient to identify parafunctional habits such as nail biting, lip and moustache sucking, pencil biting, tooth clenching, tongue and/or cheek sucking, tongue thrusting, talking without mandibular movements, and abusing soft tissue to camouflage cosmetic deficits (ie, short lips, diastemata, skeletal discrepancy, underdeveloped chin, overdeveloped nose, anatomical deviations) (see pages 62, through 64).
3. Increase self-awareness of bruxoposition. Tell the patient to place visual reminders ("stickers") in those places where he or she spends most of the day (eg, office, kitchen, car, etc) to remind him or her to stop bruxing.

4. Emphasize the importance of splint use as prescribed by the dentist (see page 64).

Abused Protrusion

Definition: A regular but abnormal posturing of the mandible in front of intercuspal position, with or without contact between the maxillary and mandibular teeth (see page 65).

Many patients with CMD have in common an abused protrusion. Abused protrusion is found in combination with several different conditions of hypermobility and bruxism. It can be recognized by the mandibular and maxillary anterior teeth in contact, as well as by a forward mandibular position without the anterior teeth in contact. Therefore it requires special attention.

The forward mandibular position encourages a forward head position. This head position is often maintained by patients exhibiting general muscle weakness and laxity. It appears that the forward mandibular position and head position encourage the increased muscle activity in the head, neck, and facial areas. This results in both pain from muscle and joint exhaustion. The patient should be taught to do the following:

1. Identify mandibular position at rest and at opening (see pages 66 and 67).
2. Recognize head posture and its relationship with the mandibular position (see pages 67 and 68).

In case the patient cannot learn to control his or her mandibular position, a stabilization splint may assist him or her in the learning process. However, most patients respond quickly when this problem is brought to their attention.

Regardless of which condition you treat, always teach and make the patient aware of the following:

1. Tongue position: Keep the tongue relaxed against the roof of the mouth.
2. Mandibular position: Keep the maxillary and mandibular teeth apart except when chewing; always rest with a small distance-space between the teeth.
3. Breathing pattern: Breathe through the nose diaphragmatically.
4. Posture positions:
   a. When standing, try to imagine a plumb line from ear to ankle through the shoulder, hip, and knee joints.
   b. When sitting, imagine a plumb line from ear to hip through the shoulder. Make sure the feet are on the ground or supported by a stool to ascertain hips and knees positioned at 90 degrees.
   c. When sleeping, position the body preferably on the back so the mandible is allowed to drop. Use a flat pillow to support the neck. If sleeping on the side, make sure that the pillow supports the vertical distance between the lateral part of the shoulder and the ear. Avoid sleeping on the stomach.
   d. When driving, maintain a proper plumb line position of sitting and make sure that the headrest is close to the back of the head. Adjust the mirrors to this position. Check the mirrors when seat-belted in this position. A lumbar support may be required to maintain this position.
5. Stress patterns: Identify and acknowledge those situations when there is a lack of control of the body. When these situations are defined, take proper steps to modify the behavior. Make sure that the patient understands and is aware of these basic rules. It is the patient's responsibility to maintain these advised conditions, otherwise physical therapy is destined to fail.

Hypermobility

Signs

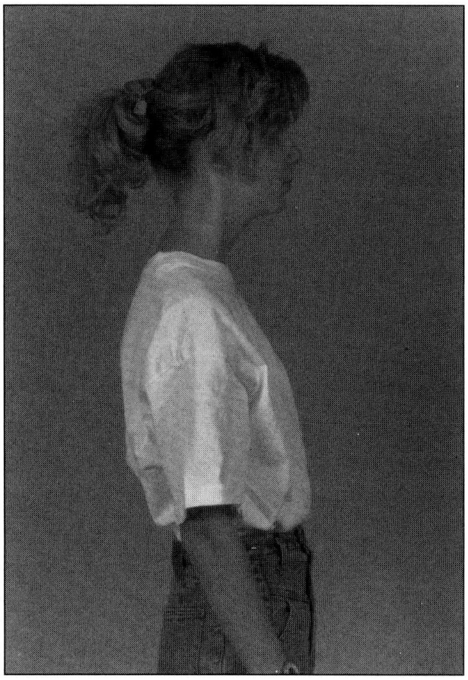

Forward head posture.

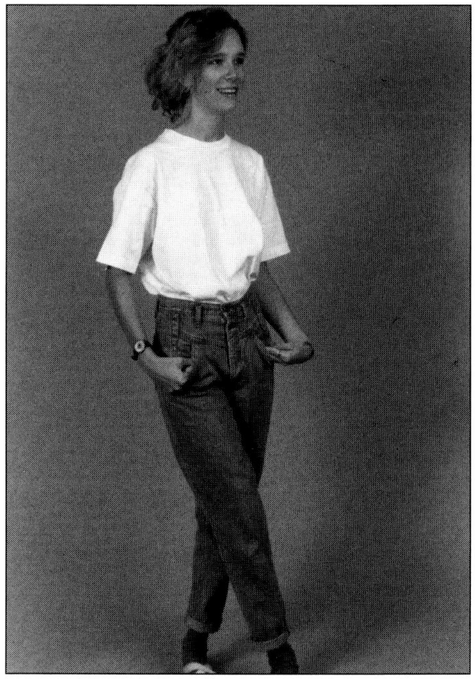

Body at rest in border position of joints.

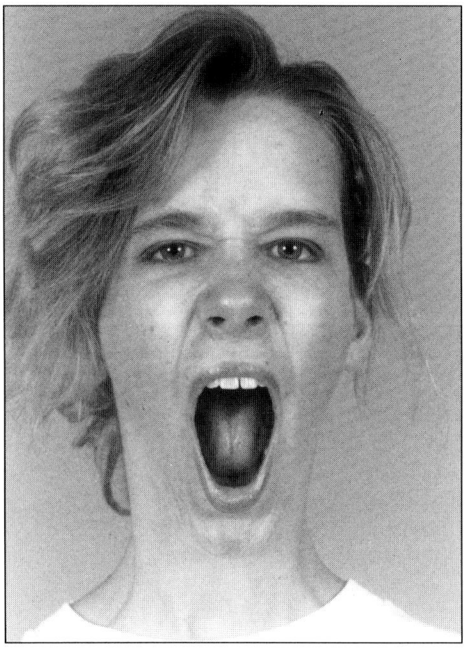

Excessive mouth opening (same patient shown on page 14, top, and on this page, top).

Hypermobility

Treatment

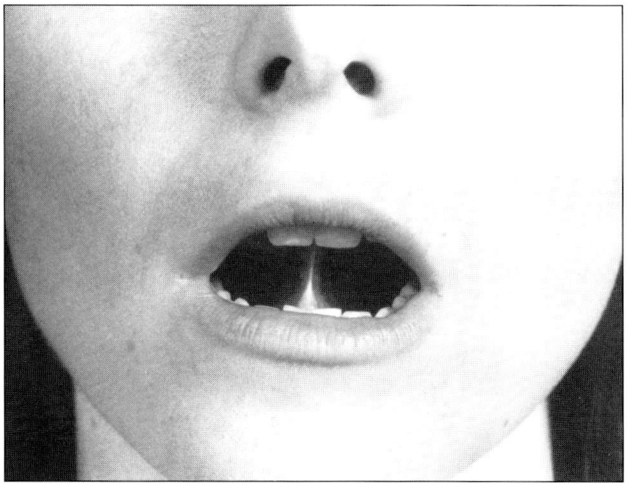
Limitation of mouth opening.

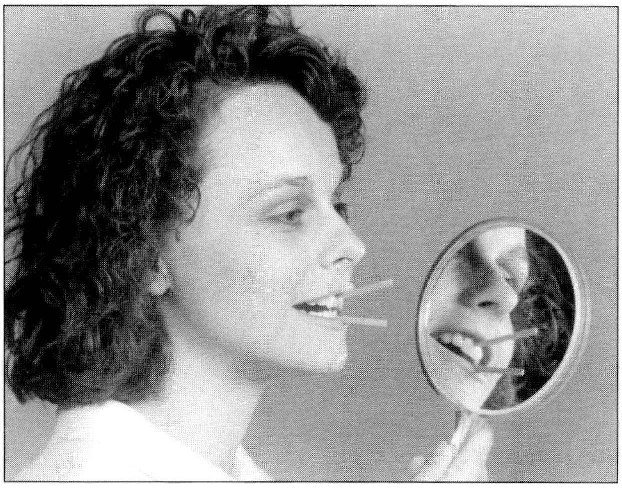
Avoidance of mandibular deviation.

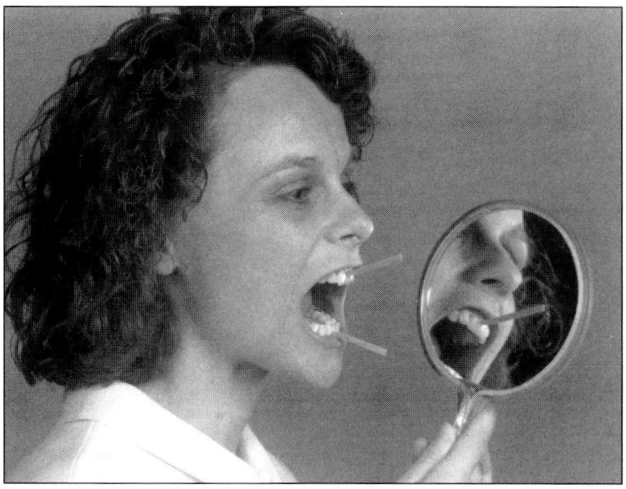
Avoidance of mandibular deviation.

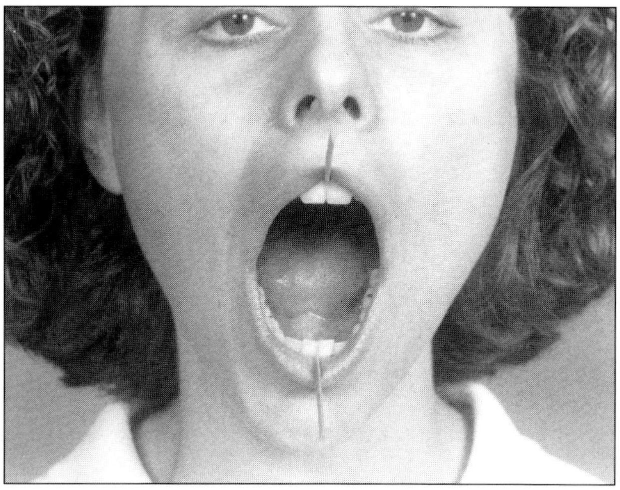
Avoidance of mandibular deviation.

Hypermobility

Treatment

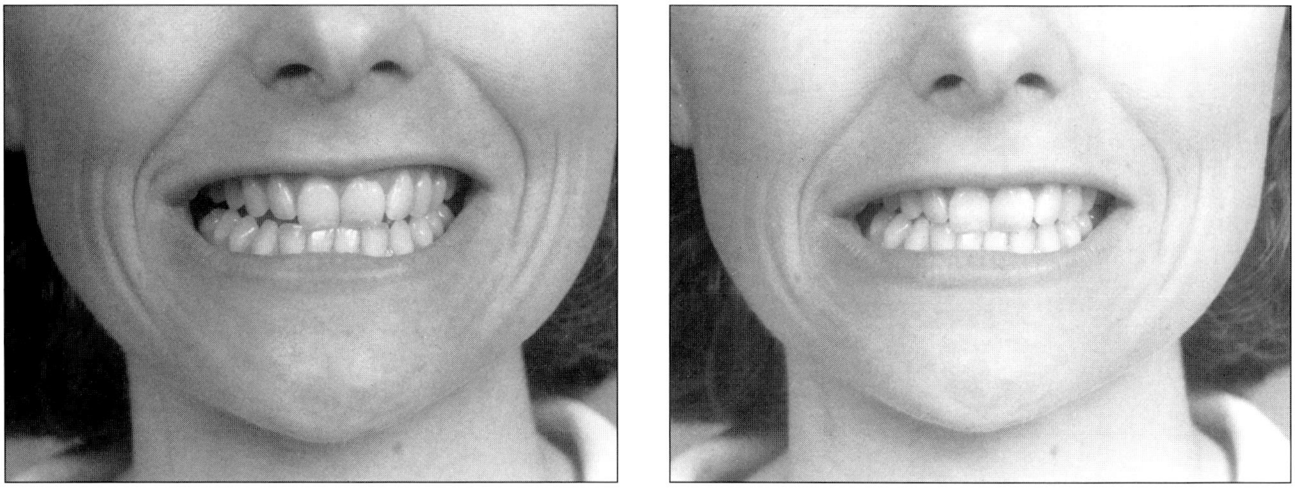

Reduce condylar translation. Emphasize condylar rotation. Avoid edge-to-edge position of the anterior teeth (frontal view).

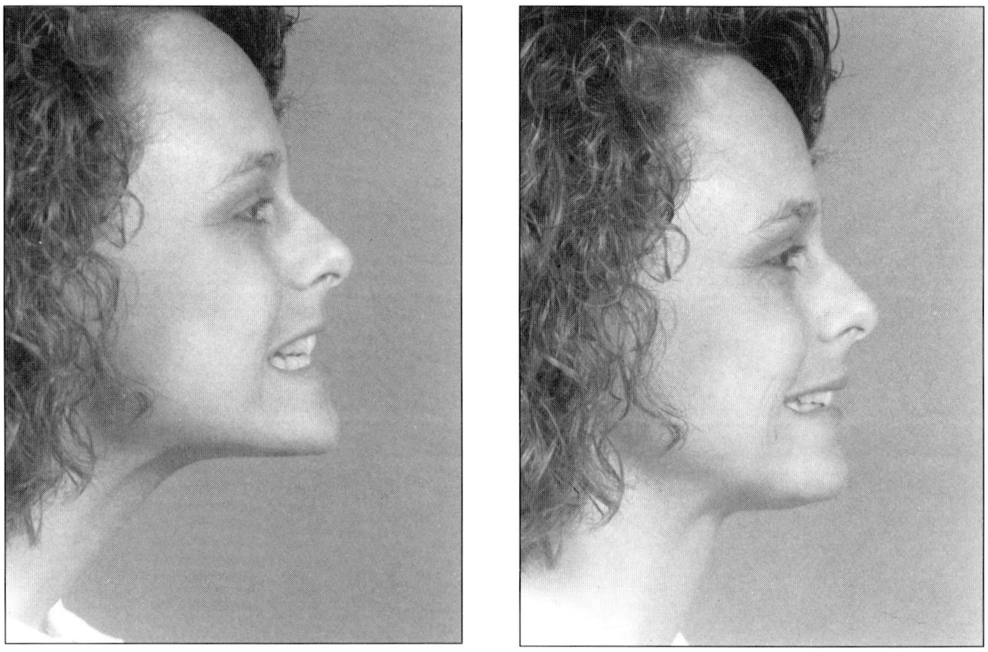

Reduce condylar translation. Emphasize condylar rotation. Avoid edge-to-edge position of the anterior teeth (sagittal view).

Hypermobility

Treatment

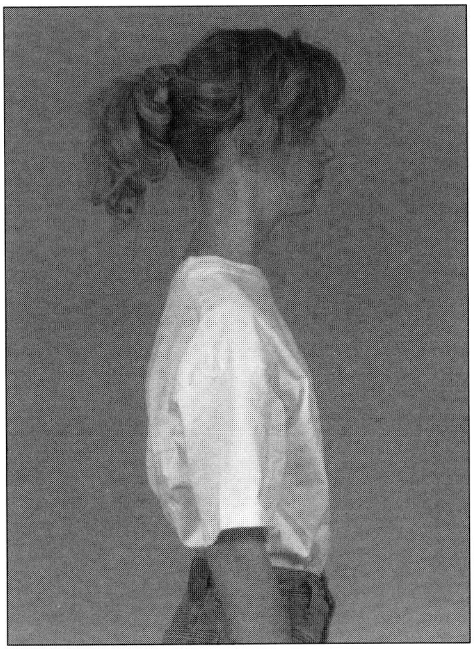

Improve head posture (compare with previous posture position; see page 46, top left).

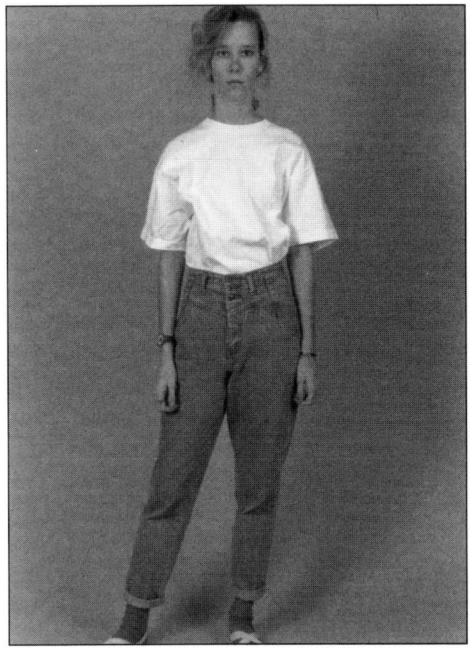

Improve body posture (compare with previous posture position; see page 46, top right).

Hypermobility

Treatment

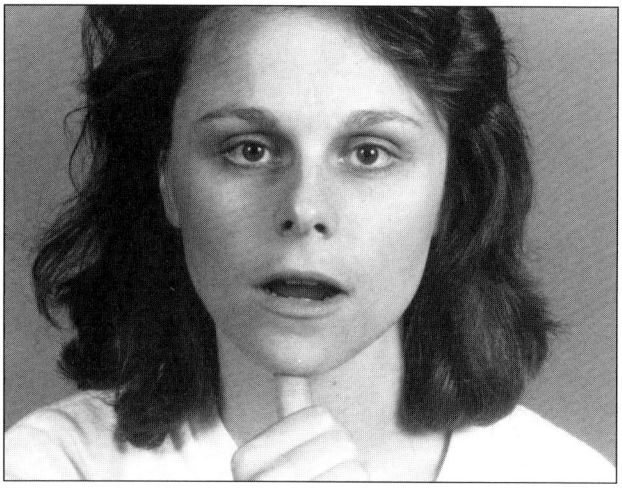

Resist manually active mandibular movements. Mouth opening.

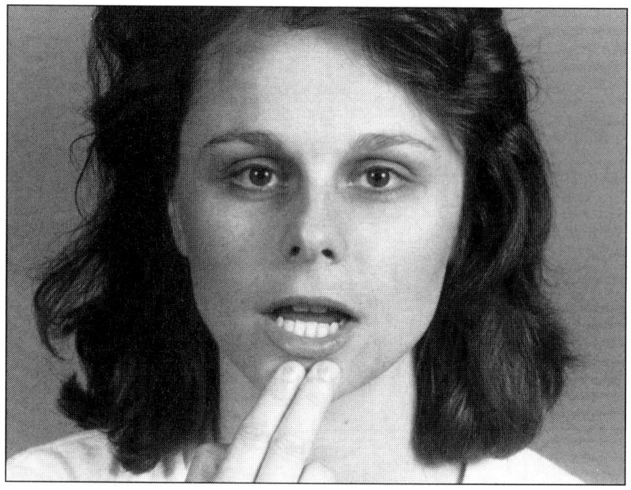

Resist manually active mandibular movements. Protrusion. Do not apply to patients who have abused protrusion.

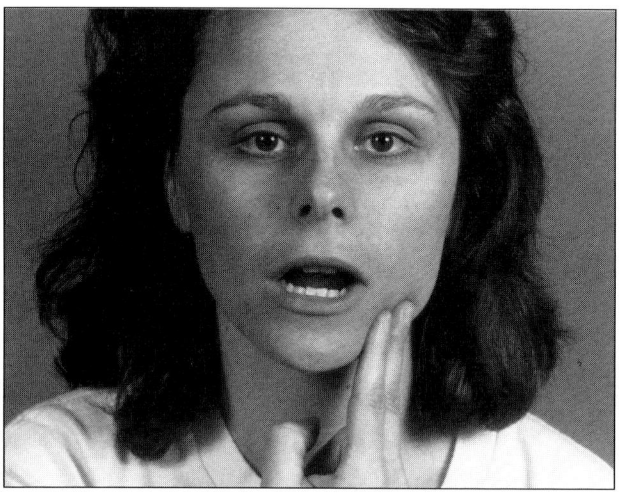

Resist manually active mandibular movements. Laterotrusion to the left.

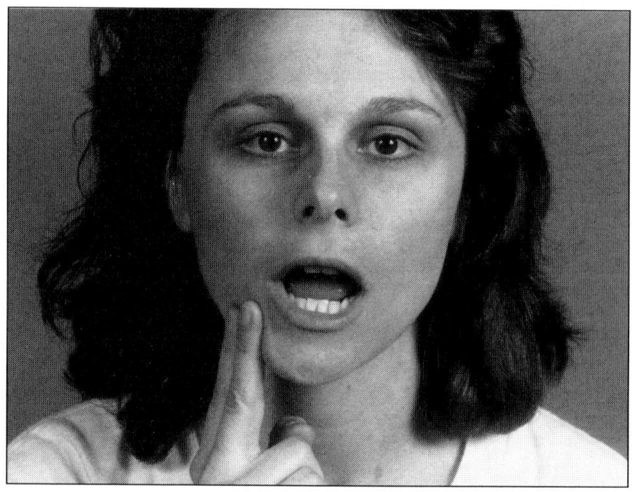

Resist manually active mandibular movements. Laterotrusion to the right.

Hypermobility

Treatment

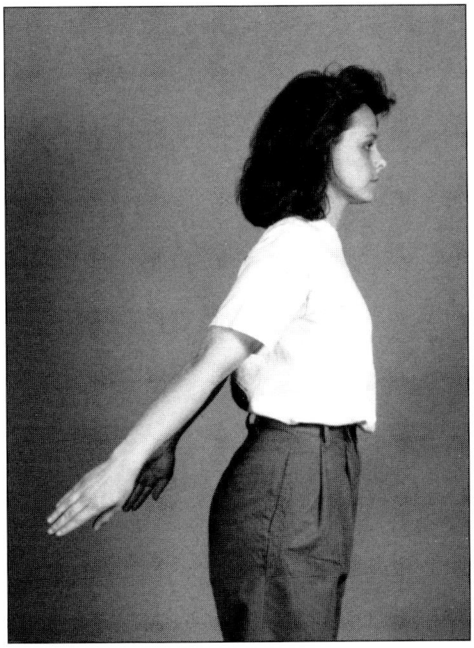

Shoulder extension.

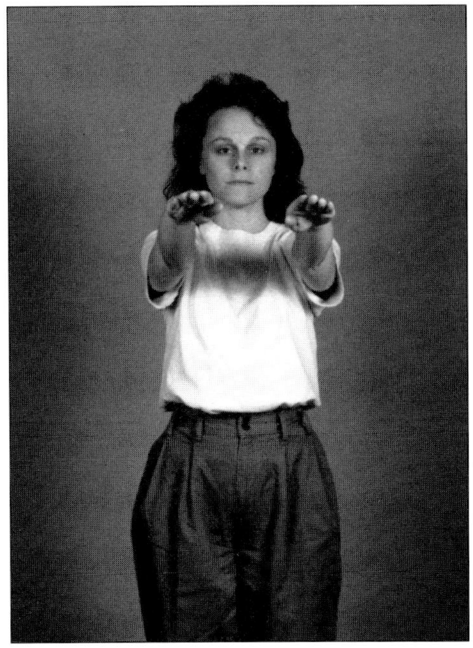

Shoulder flexion.

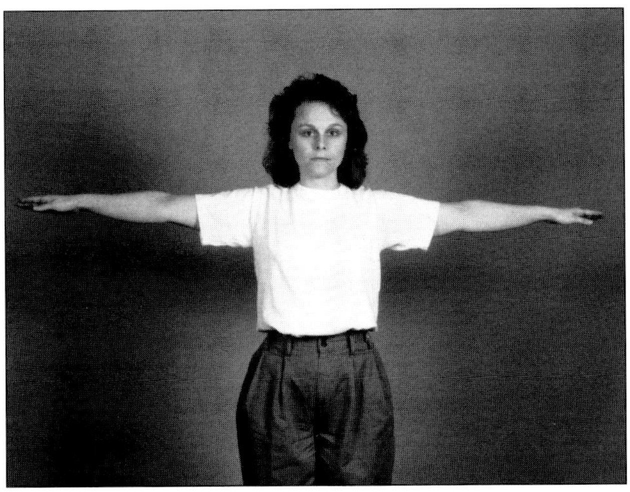

Shoulder abduction.

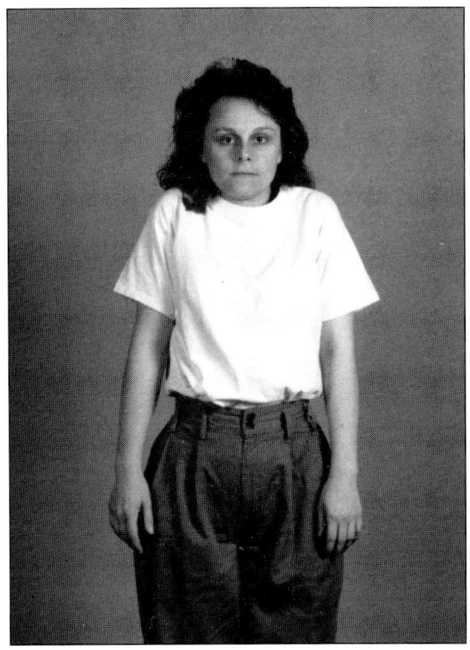

Shoulder elevation–shrug.

Hypermobility

Treatment

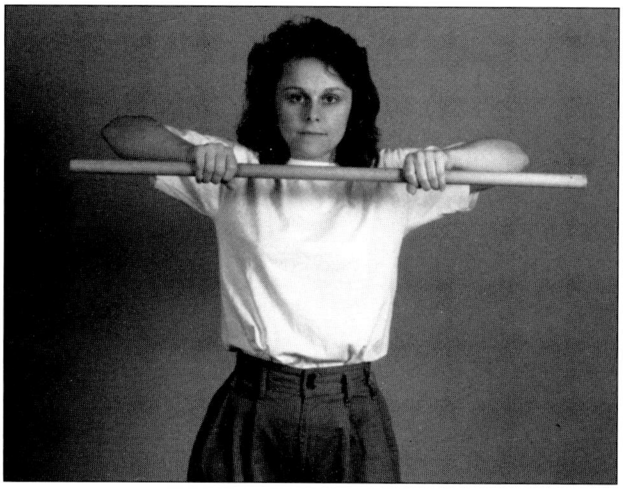

Shoulder abduction with internal rotation. Upright rows.

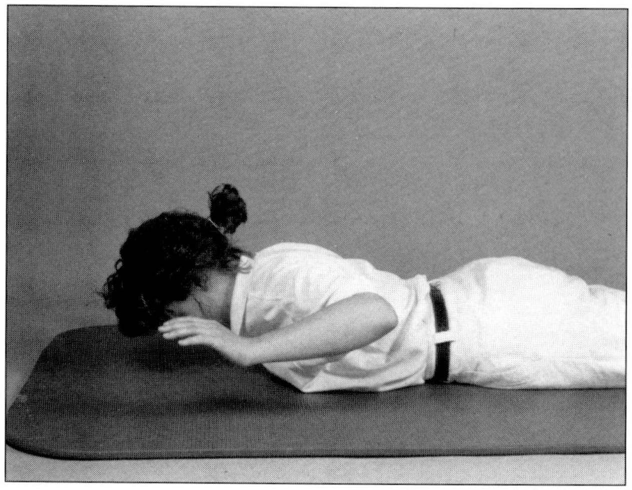

Scapular muscles, trunk and neck extensors.

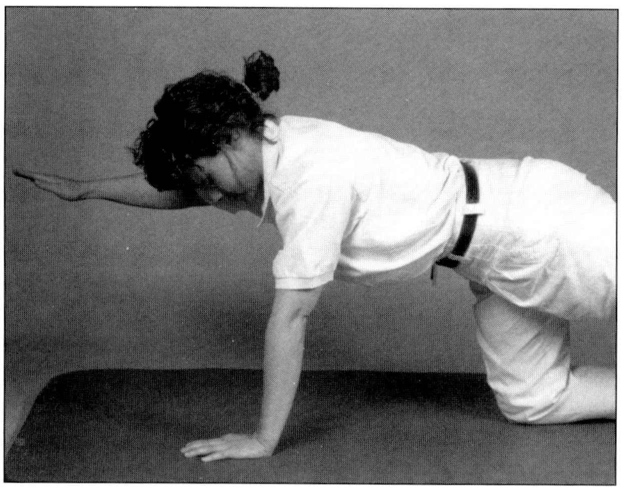

Neck, trunk and hip extensors.

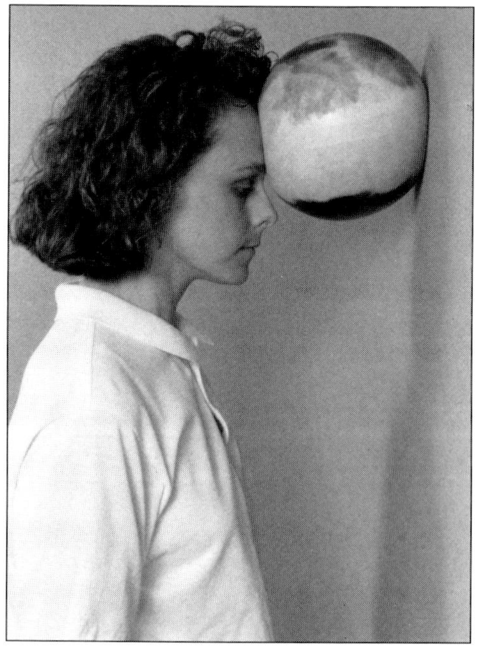

Cervical flexion. Maintain a proper posture. Use the "ball on the wall" as a resistance for strengthening the muscles.

Hypermobility

Treatment

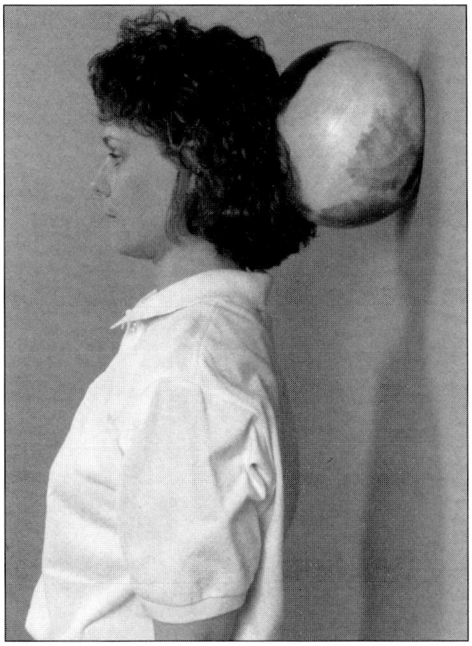

Cervical extension. Maintain a proper posture. Use the "ball on the wall" as a resistance for strengthening the muscles.

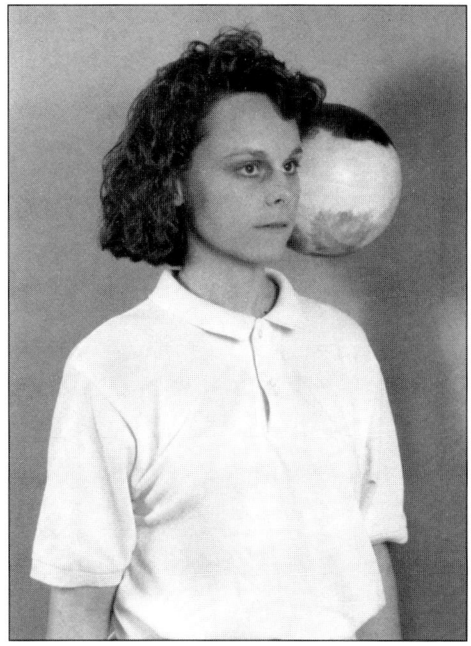

Cervical rotation. Maintain a proper posture. Use the "ball on the wall" as a resistance for strengthening the muscles.

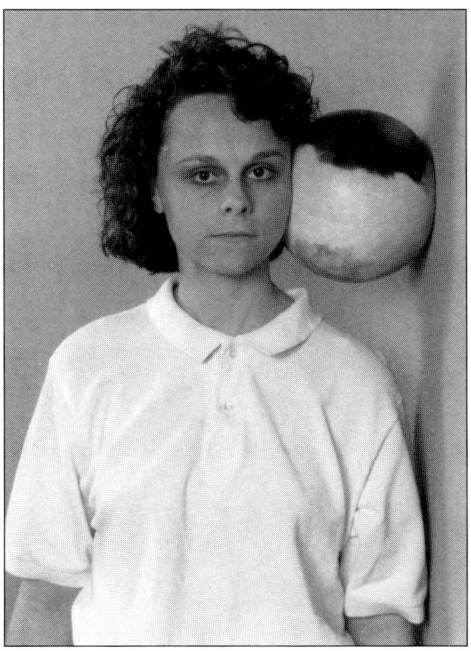

Cervical lateroflexion. Maintain a proper posture. Use the "ball on the wall" as a resistance for strengthening the muscles.

Hypomobility

Signs

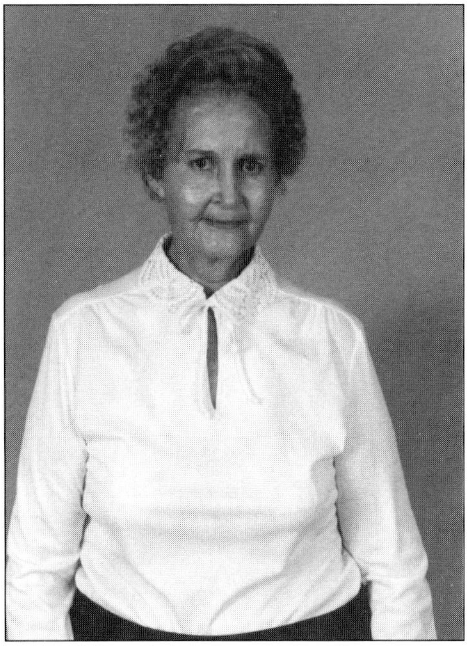

Facial tightness.

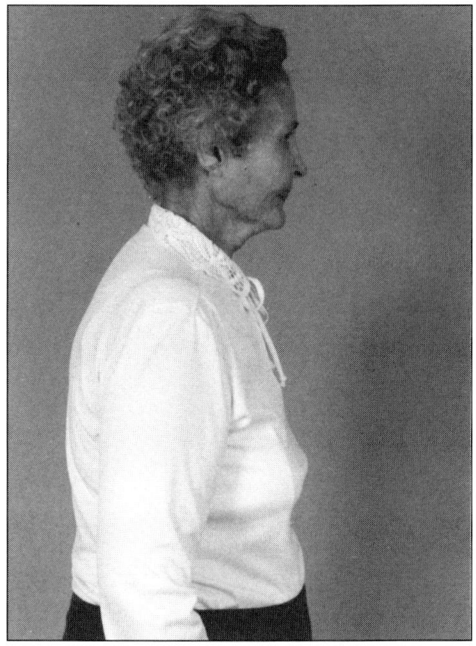

Rigid posture.

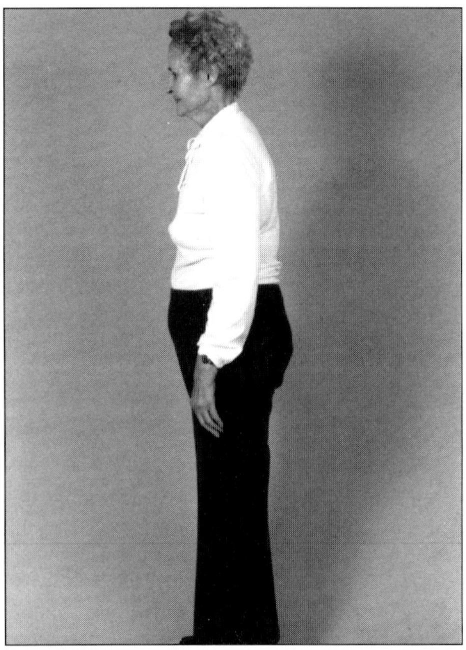

Rigid posture.

Hypomobility

Treatment

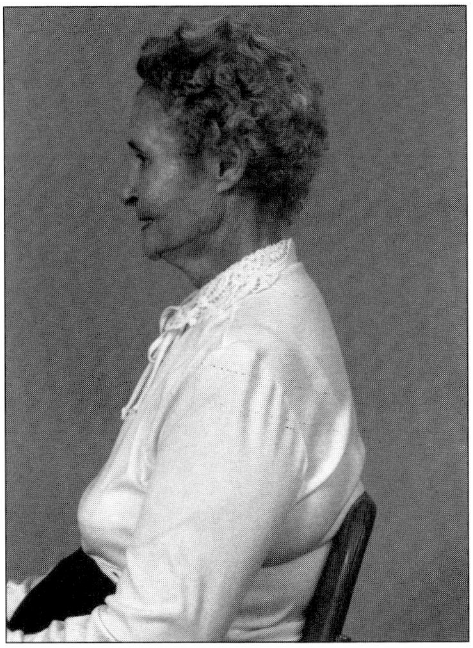

Exaggerate mandibular rest. Emphasize a loose, hanging mandible.

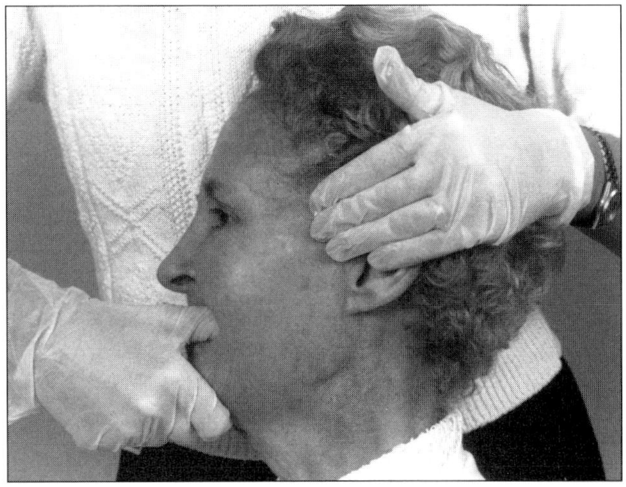

Perform manual traction and translation (see page 39).

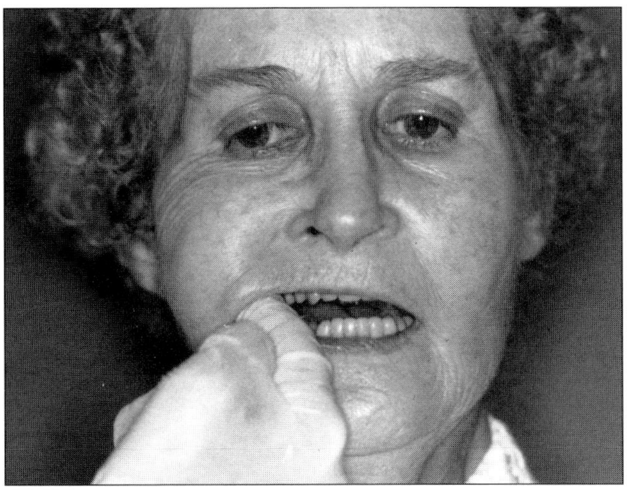

Perform and instruct manual muscular stretching. Start at the origin of the masseter muscle in the area of the zygomatic arch.

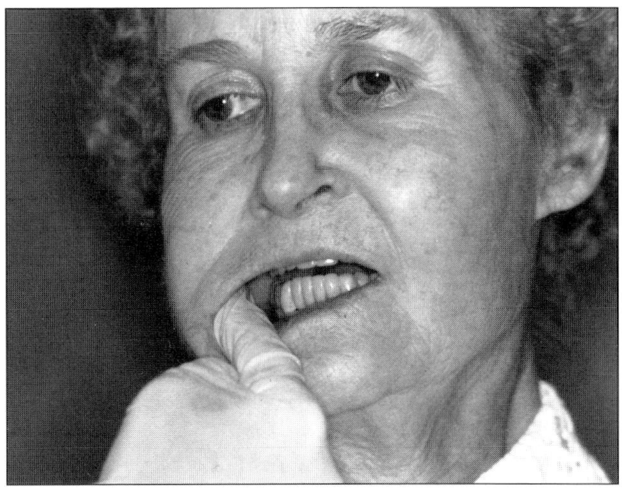

Perform manual muscular stretching. Make sure to reach and sweep the whole belly of the masseter muscle.

Hypomobility

Treatment

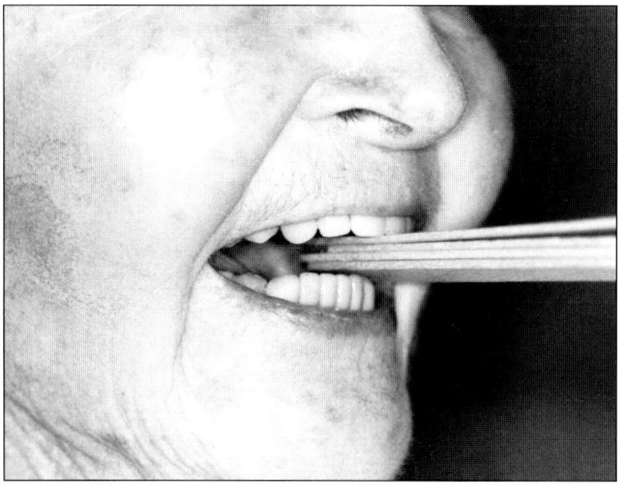

Use assistive devices (eg, tongue blades). Motivate to increase the amount of tongue blades used from time to time.

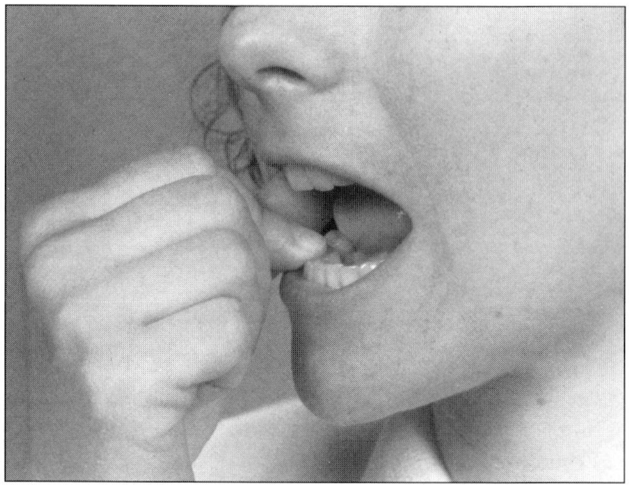

Put the thumb on the edges of the maxillary teeth and the index or the long finger on the edges of the mandibular teeth. Apply force against the teeth.

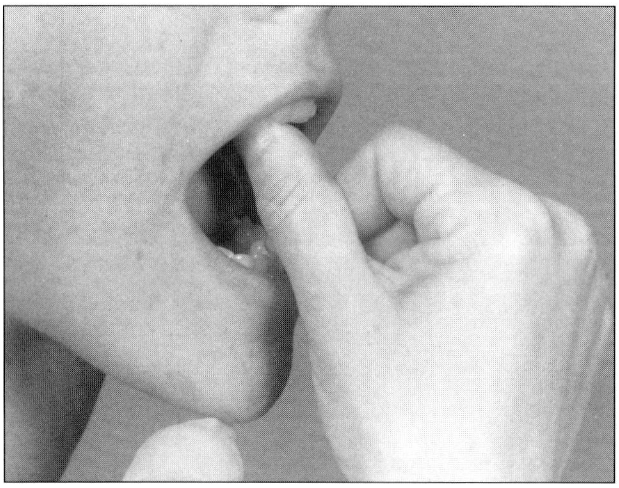

Encourage patient participation.

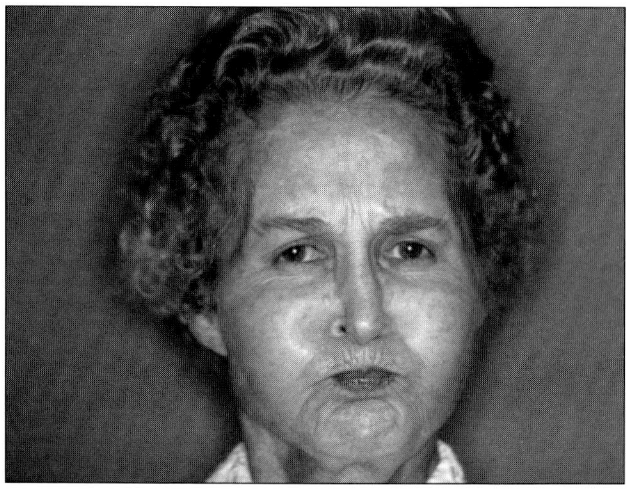

Hold air in the cheeks. Move the air from side to side.

Hypomobility

Treatment

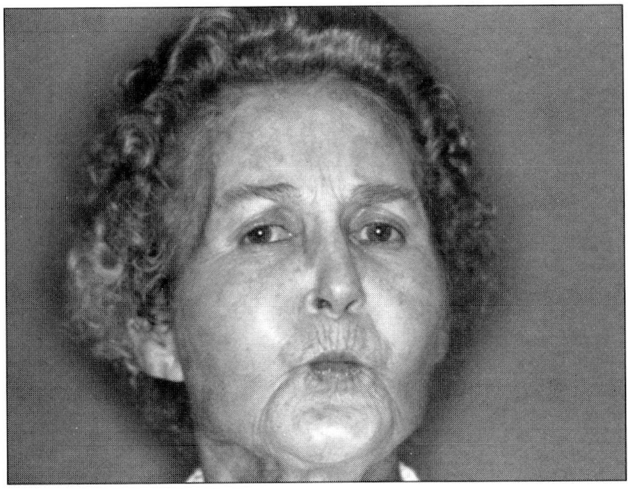

Compress the lips and pucker.

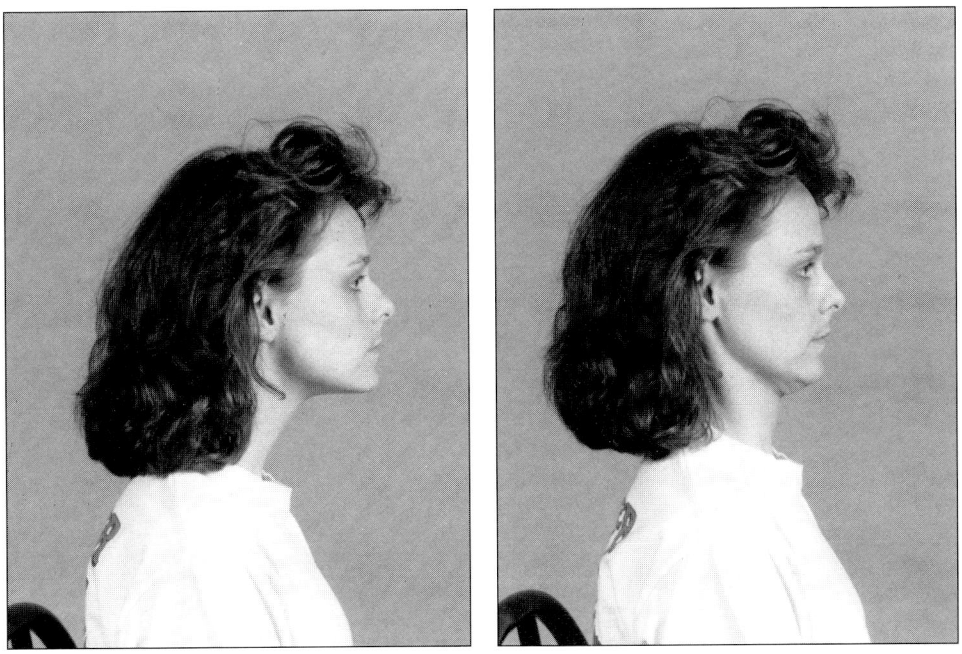

Move into axial extension.

Hypomobility

Treatment

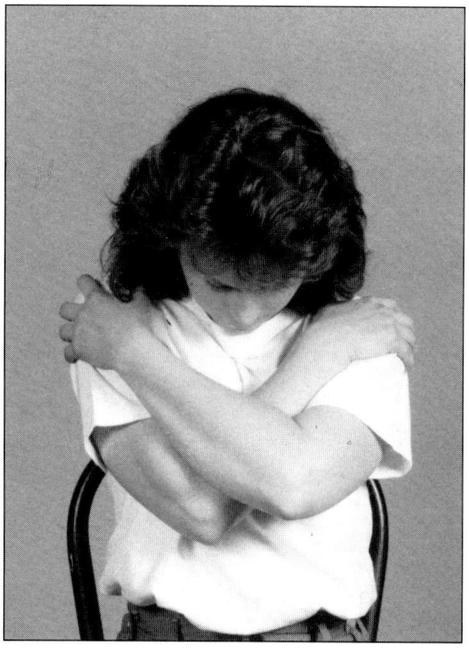

Flexion with arms crossed and chin tucked.

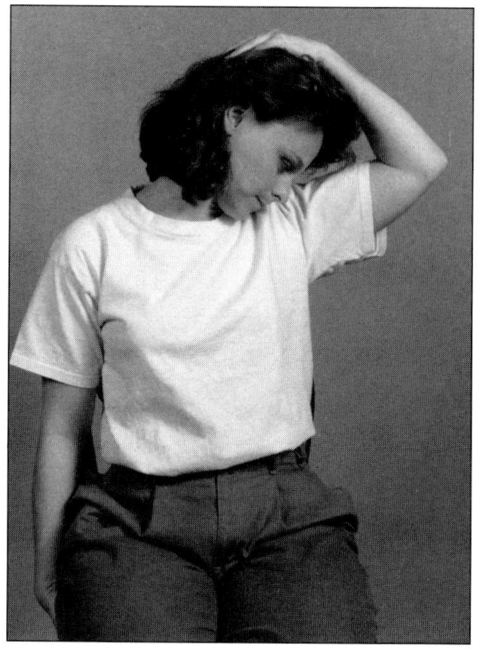

Cervical rotation and flexion.

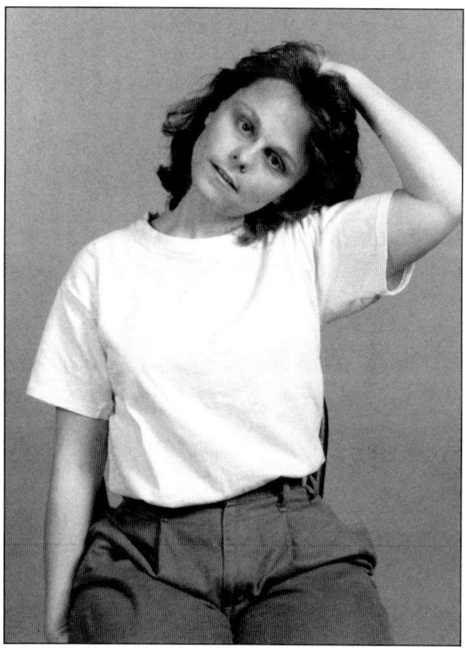

Lateroflexion.

Hypomobility

Treatment

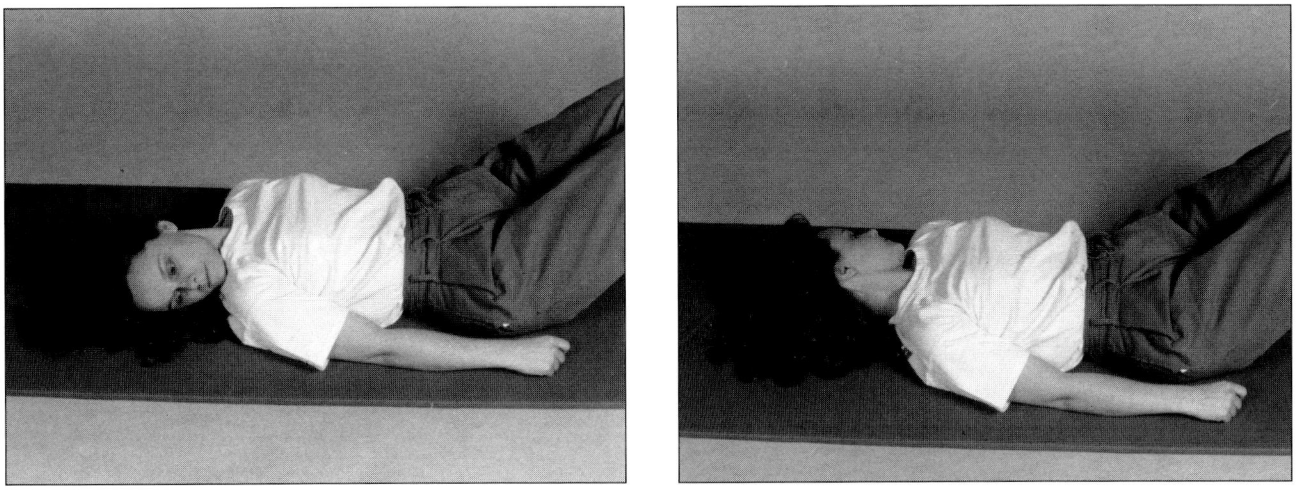

Supine position, cervical rotation. Do not lift the head.

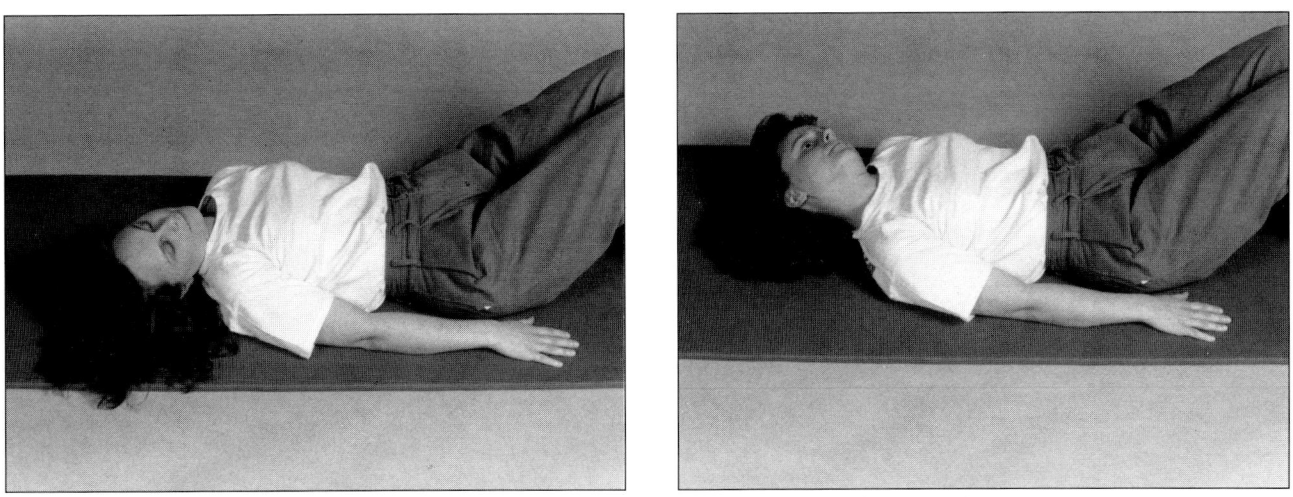

Supine position, cervical lateroflexion. Do not lift the head.

Hypomobility

Treatment

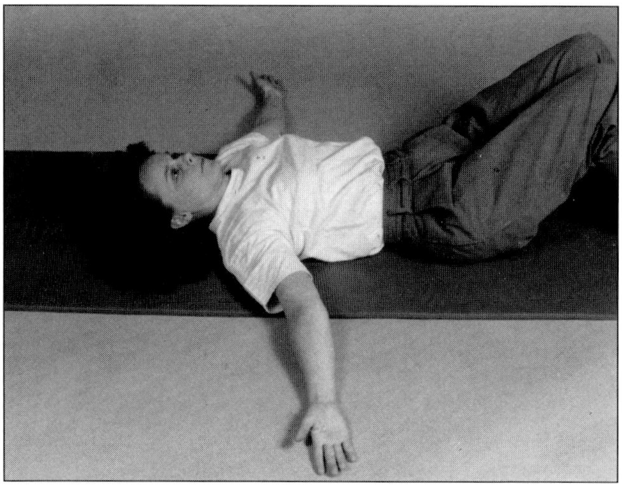
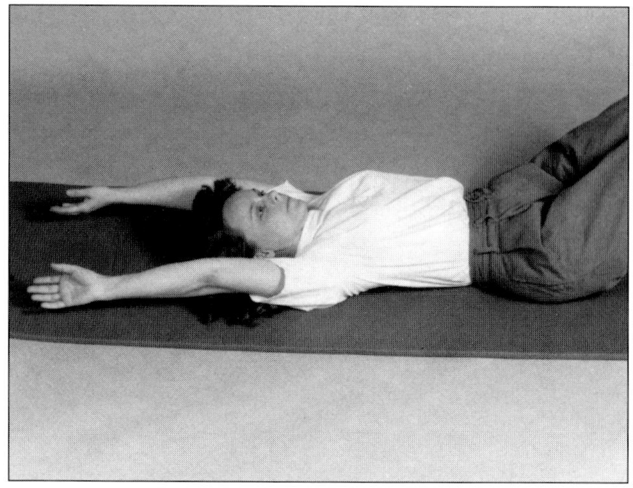

Shoulder abduction. Keep the arms in contact with the surface and raise them above the head.

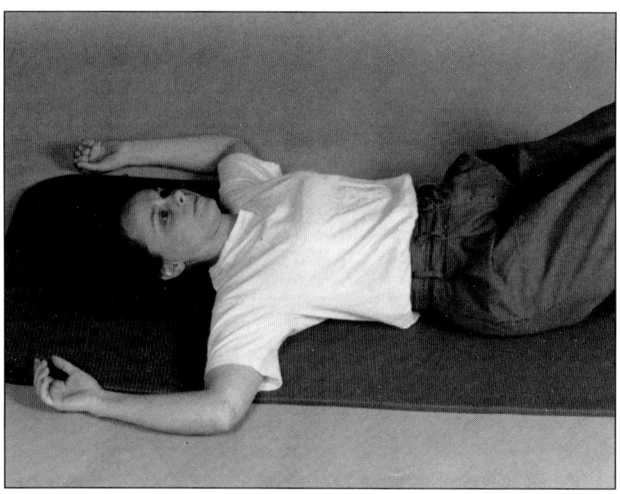
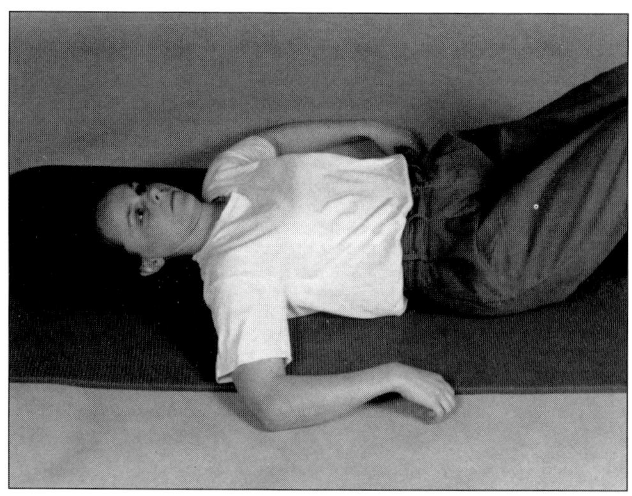

Shoulder rotation. Keep the upper part of the arm in contact with the surface.

Bruxism

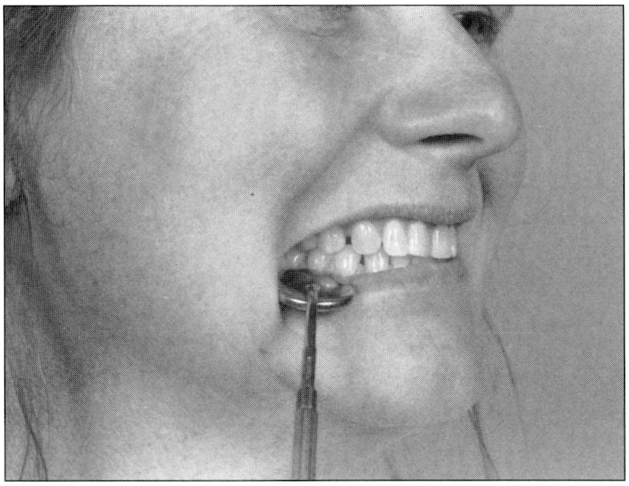

Continuous contact between the teeth: clenching.

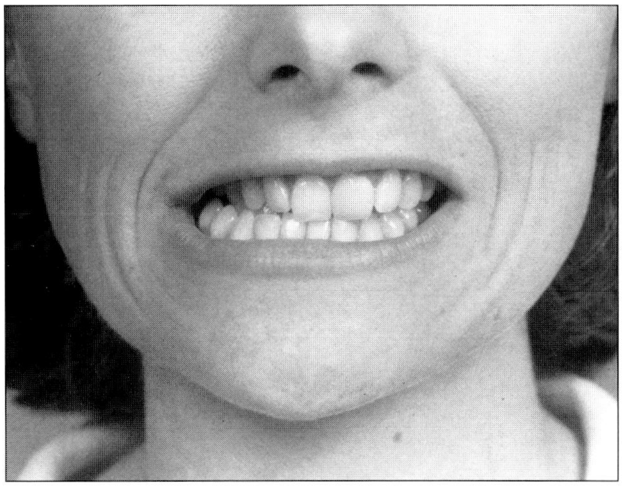

Contact between some teeth during continuous mandibular movement: grinding.

Bruxism

Bruxism with Additional Parafunction

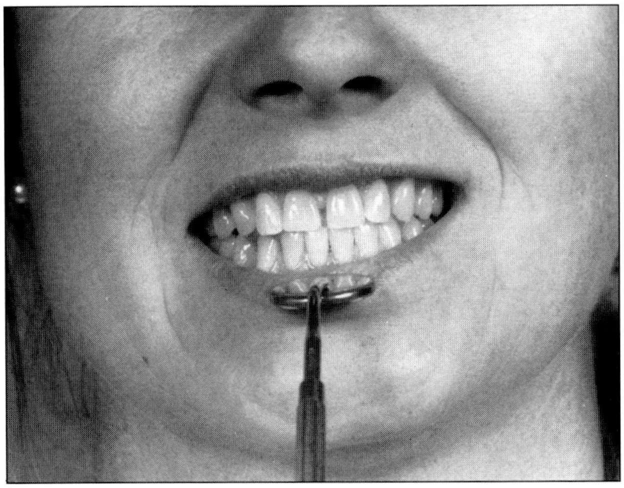

Continuous pressure of the tongue against the teeth with or without clenching-grinding.

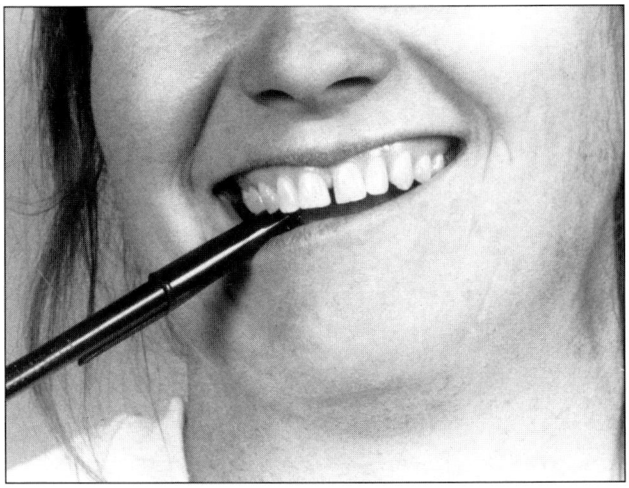

Continuous pressure against some teeth with a foreign object.

Bruxism

"Treatment"

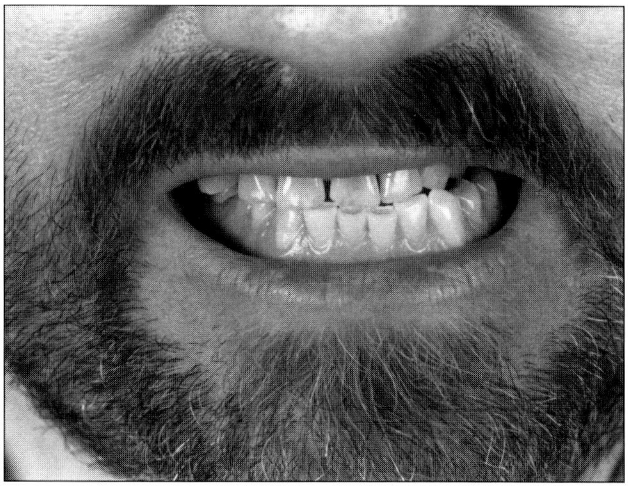

Location of bruxo facets. Identify the facets between the anterior teeth for improper wear to increase the patient's awareness.

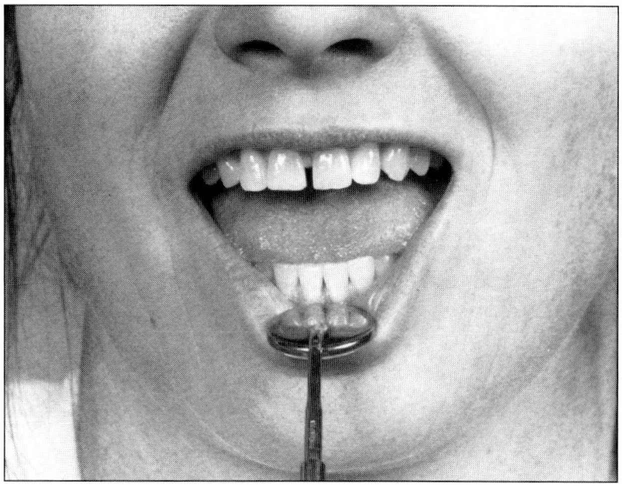

Location of bruxo facets. Identify the facets between the anterior teeth for improper wear to increase the patient's awareness. Minor facets are made easily visible when teeth are dry.

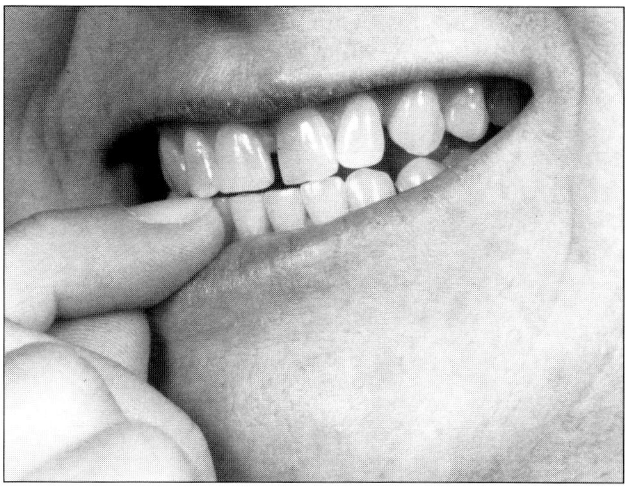

Explain the negative effects of nail biting regarding the dental wear due to the abrasive nature of the nail between the teeth and the repetitive mandibular position.

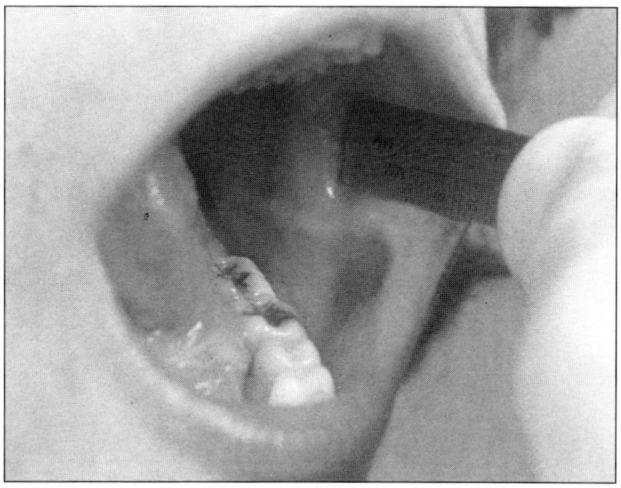

Cheek sucking. Identify and increase the patient's awareness of the soft tissue buildup of the inner surface of the cheek at the level of the occlusal plane.

Bruxism

"Treatment"

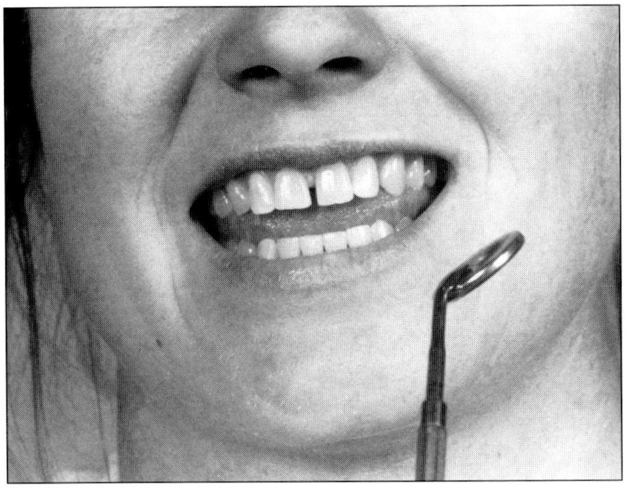

Tongue sucking. Identify and increase the patient's awareness of impressions of the lingual surfaces of the teeth on the tongue border.

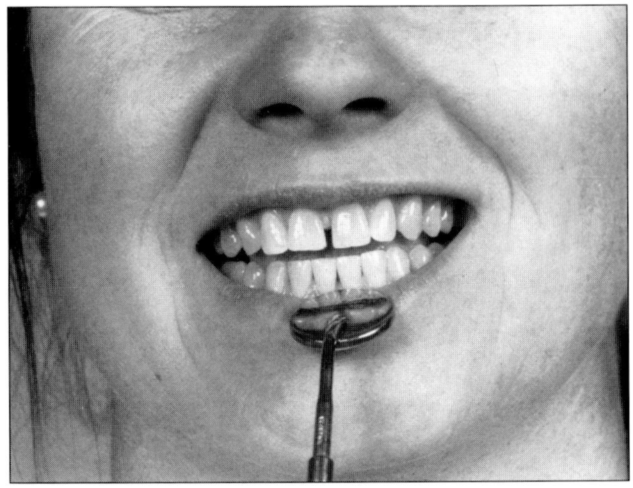

Tongue sucking. Identify and increase the patient's awareness of how the tongue occupies the distance between the maxillary and mandibular teeth at rest.

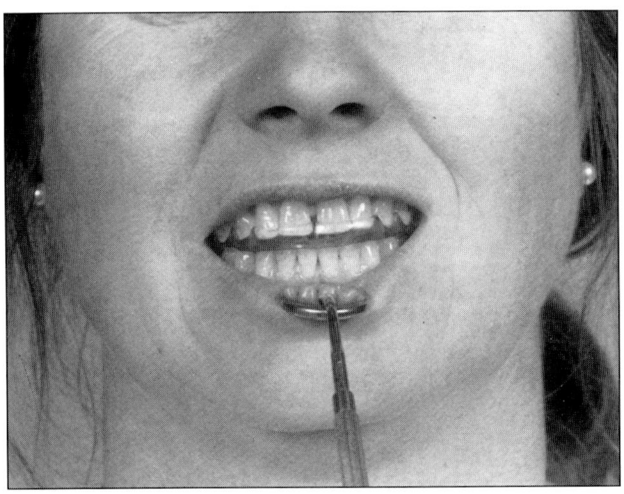

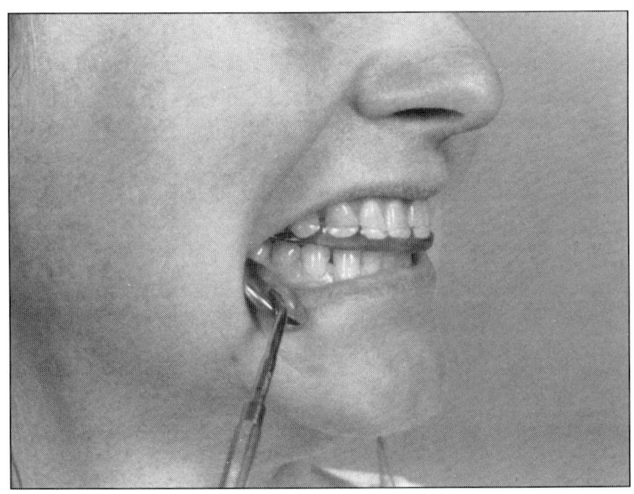

Splint. The patient should keep the splint available for those occasions when he or she will be unable to control bruxing habits.

Abused Protrusion

Signs

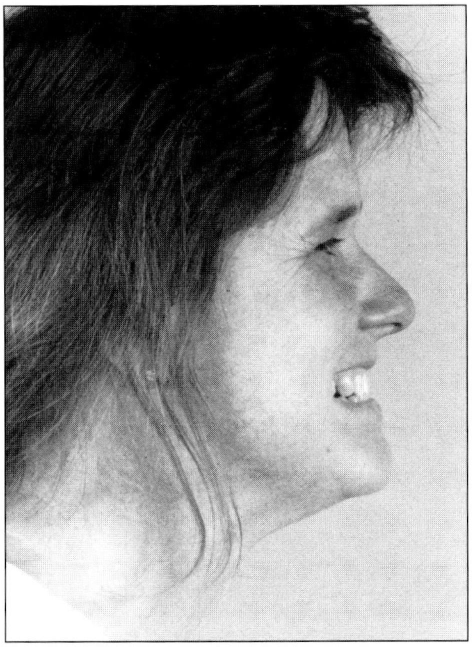

Mandibular protrusion with the maxillary and mandibular anterior teeth in contact.

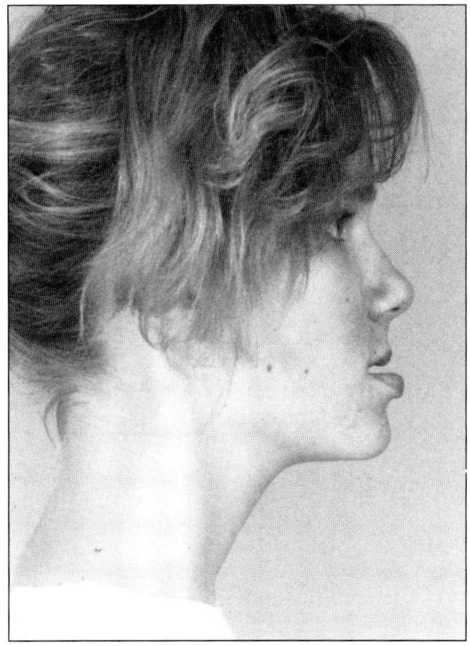

Mandibular protrusion without tooth contact.

Abused Protrusion

"Treatment"

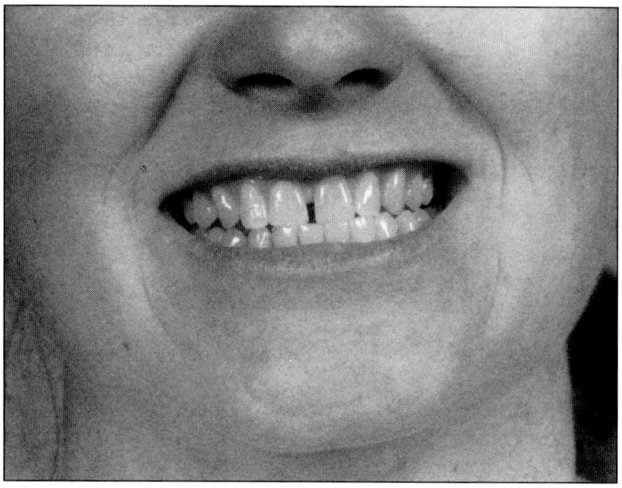

Identify the improper rest position and increase patient's awareness of its effects on muscles, joints, and teeth (frontal view).

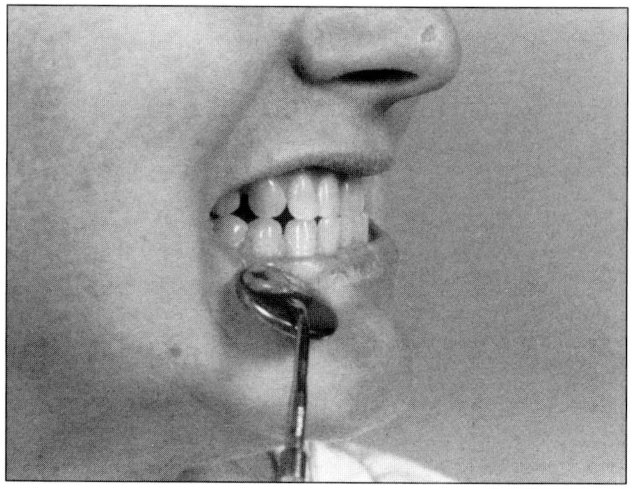

Identify the improper rest position and increase patient's awareness of its effects on muscles, joints, and teeth (sagittal view).

Abused Protrusion

"Treatment"

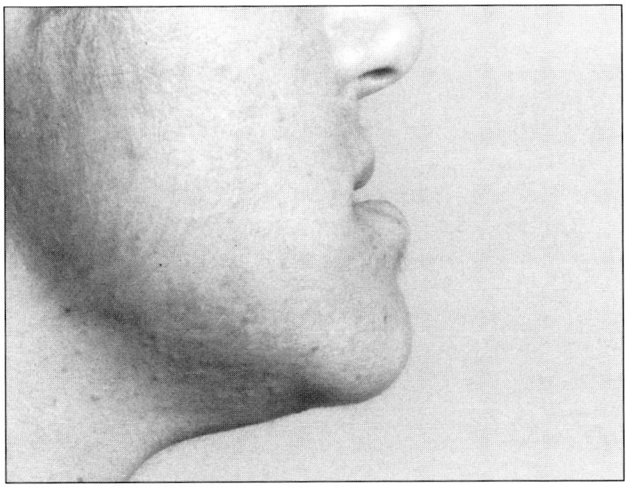

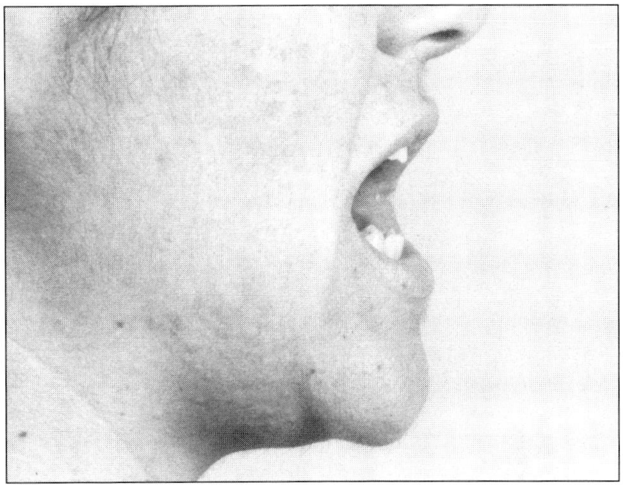

Identify and show the patient when his or her mandible is pushed forward during the initial phases of mouth opening.

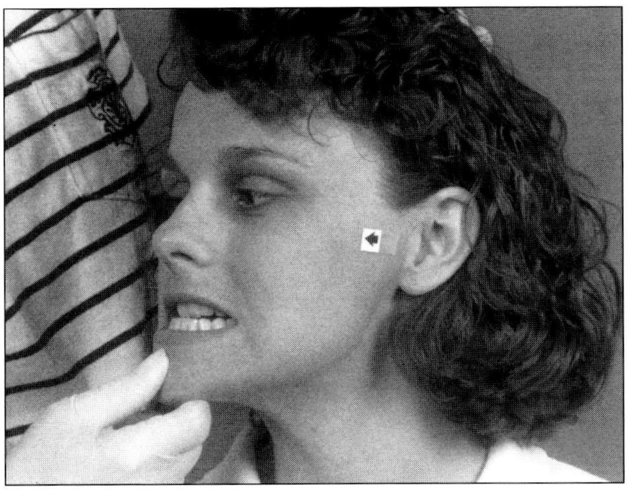

Identify and increase the patient's awareness of the forward head posture with the forward mandibular rest position.

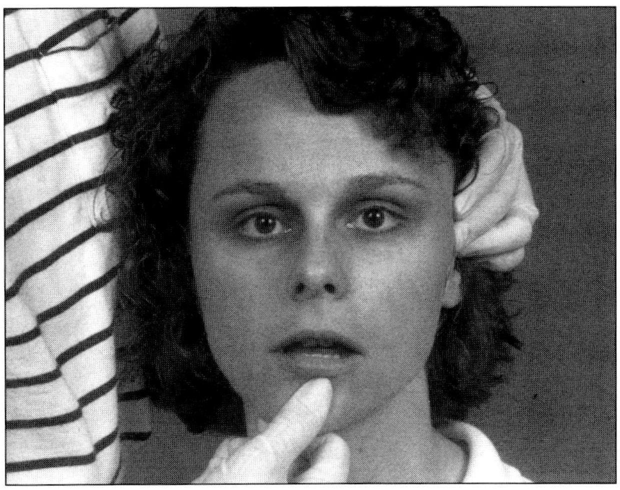

Identify and explain the proper TMJ condyle-disc complex behavior at rest and on mouth opening.

Abused Protrusion

"Treatment"

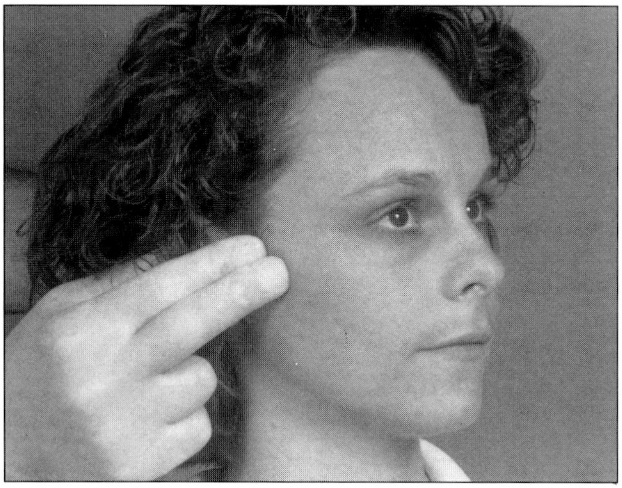

Identify and demonstrate the TMJ behavior at rest. Avoid anterior teeth contact or a forward position of the mandible.

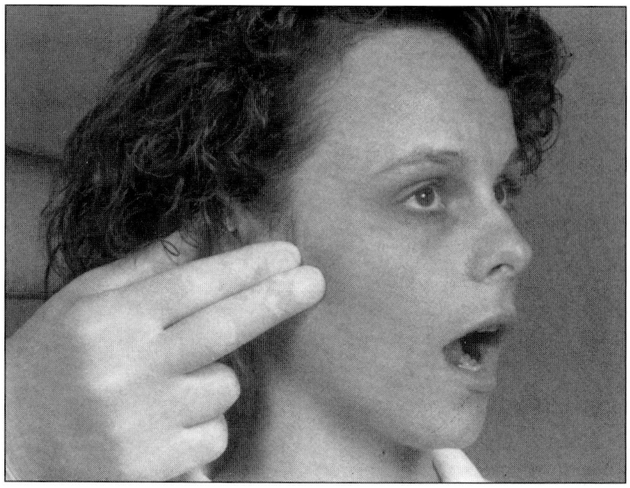

Identify and demonstrate the TMJ behavior to mid mouth opening. Emphasize the importance of TMJ condylar rotation. Avoid TMJ condylar translation.

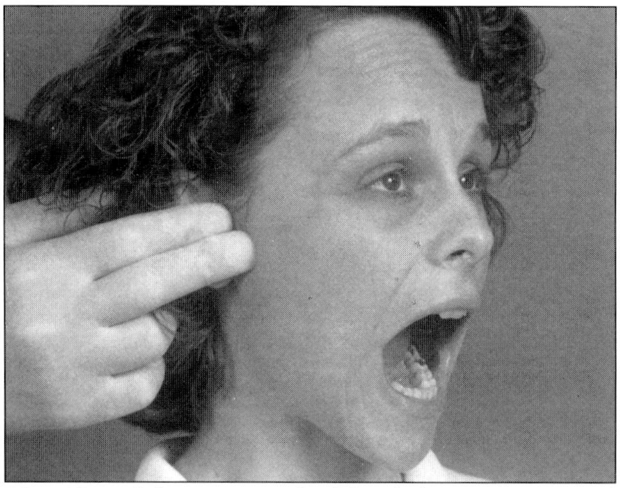

Identify and demonstrate the TMJ behavior at maximal mouth opening. Avoid any forward movement of the mandible. When terminal TMJ clicking occurs at the end of mouth opening, advise the patient to decrease mouth opening.

Problems

4

Some conditions of the TMJ need special attention from a physiotherapeutical point of view. Definite joint pathology diagnosed as (1) anterior displacement of the TMJ disc without reduction, (2) postoperative TMJ pain, (3) osteoarthrosis, and (4) acute TMJ arthritis must be handled with utmost consideration.

Anterior Displacement of the TMJ Disc Without Reduction

This is recognized by the deviation of the chin to the affected side with limited mouth opening. Side movements of the mandible are asymmetrical with a clear reduction of laterotrusion to the contralateral side. When the mandible is brought forward (ie, protrusion), the chin also deviates to the affected side. The clinical situation may resemble a muscular problem. However, the clinical history indicates whether a TMJ clicking sound has been present in the past. If so, the articular situation can be explained by the probable fact of long-lasting intra-articular overloading. Soft tissue irregularities of the joint surfaces with or without a proper disc alignment have reduced the potential for continuing biomechanics of translation. The disc is positioned in front of the condyle and is from one second to the next an impediment for translation. This condition most often occurs unilaterally. It is an effect of unilateral overloading or clenching with or without a morphological reason. The clinical picture of unilateral deviation on opening and protrusion is therefore easy to understand and should prohibit the physical therapist from manipulative exercises. If stretching is applied to such a joint, the risk for perforation of the posterior ligaments is very likely.

Any treatment of this condition must aim at the maintenance of the condyle in its posterior position. Thus, rotational condylar movements are the only ones to emphasize. Translation is to be avoided with training of the rotational movements. An opening capacity of the mouth is achievable in the range of 30 to 40 mm.

Postoperative Pain

This must be recognized as the result of a posttraumatic condition. The inflammatory reaction needs to be monitored by the oral surgeon, dentist, or physician. Intensive dosages of anti-inflammatory medication is the most efficient treatment. No physiotherapeutic exercises are recommended until the inflammation is resolved.

Osteoarthrosis

Osteoarthrosis is recognized by the TMJ sound of crepitation. This sound is produced by rough and degenerated joint surfaces articulating against each other. The arthrotic lesion is a sign of local exhaustion of adaptation of the joint component. The reserve of undifferentiated mesenchymal cells is exhausted. Although the joint noises are audible and most often magnified by the resonance of the bony environment, the very lesion inside the joint is small. Therefore, it is possible to avoid the region of the lesion, which most often is the result of adverse loading in one and the same mandibular position. Rotational movements need to be emphasized in the physiotherapeutic sessions. The main part of the program is to break the oral habit that is the cause for overloading the system.

Acute TMJ Arthritis

An acute arthritis is found as the immediate response to a trauma. This immediate inflammatory reaction compulsively changes the total behavior of the surrounding muscles. The initial part of physical therapy should not be focused on the changes of muscle function. Utmost care must therefore be given to trauma cases. If time is given to the resolution of the intra-articular inflammation, the muscle function will also return to normal. Anti-inflammatory medication combined with information about the preceding events should be the only treatment given within the first 1 or 2 weeks after the trauma. Changes of occlusion are absolutely prohibited.

During these four conditions we have mentioned, the dentist needs to be in charge of the treatment otherwise treatment will fail. Any physiotherapeutical exercise not aimed at the maintenance of the condylar position within the temporal component risks aggravating the condition.

Recent studies on the effect of the applications of infrared (IR) laser at the arthrogenous origin of pain indicate the beneficial effect of reduction of inflammation at an energy level applied at 100 MJ/session (Bezuur et al, 1988c; Hansson 1989; Hansson 1990). However the infrared light will not permanently eliminate the inflammation if it is not combined with occlusal stability. Therefore, when application of IR laser is indicated, it should be given in conjunction with dental treatment aimed at occlusal stability. Until further scientific results are published, IR laser when applied as described is only an alternative for reducing intra-articular inflammation.

Conclusion

5

This book addressed the pure mechanical corrections for determined unilateral overloading of the stomatognathic system. When physical therapy is prescribed, the patient should be informed about the reason for the referral by the dentist. Included in the planning should be the time needed to accomplish the change of habit that may cause or be a contributing factor to the reaction of pain. Within the predetermined time, the patient should have subjective awareness of improvement. The plan of treatment should be structured at the initial visit with the dentist. Additional information and timing of treatment should be given by the physical therapist when the training sessions start.

The patient should be actively involved in the treatment with the emphasis at first on posture, stretching, and strengthening. If symptoms do not decrease, other modalities may be necessary. As the patient acknowledges his or her improvement during the regular and predetermined sessions, there will be a decrease in the need for physical therapy and longer intervals between therapy sessions are acceptable. This schedule allows the physical therapist to be in command during a longer period of time, although the patient is the most active member, through awareness and daily exercises in the home environment, of the pain-reducing team.

Appendix. Physical Therapy Examination Protocol

St. Joseph's Hospital
and Medical Center
Outpatient Physical Therapy

PATIENT'S SELF ASSESSMENT

NAME: ______________________ PATIENT NUMBER ______________

AGE: ______ TODAY'S DATE __________ YOUR DIAGNOSIS ______________

REFERRING DOCTOR/DENTIST ______________ OCCUPATION: ______________

Briefly describe your present problem in your own words (e.g., pain, numbness, weakness, etc.):

____

____

When did your problem begin and how did your problem start? ______________

____

____

If this is an on-going problem, when did it worsen? ______________

What treatment have you had so far (or are you presently receiving)? ______________

____

____

PAIN: ☐ Constant ☐ Intermittent (comes and goes)

Aggravated/worsened by: ______________

Relieved by: ______________

Location: Please use the pain drawing and codes to show where your pain is.

= sharp

= shooting

= tightness/dull pain

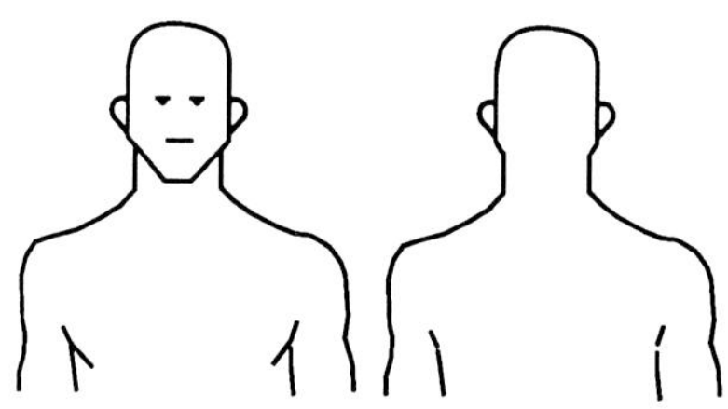

Intensity: Please rate your pain on the following scale (0 = no pain, 10 = worst imaginable pain):

0 1 2 3 4 5 6 7 8 9 10

FUNCTION: Please list any activities that you are now unable to do because of your present problem:

____

____

Feel free to give any other information related to your problem: ______________

____

Do you have any medical problems? ______________

____

Are you under a doctor's care for any problem other than what we are seeing you for?

____

____

OPD-2076

CERVICAL EVALUATION

Patient Name ____________________

Patient Number ____________________

POSTURE:

Forward head: ____________________ Rounded shoulders: ____________________

Kyphotic: ____________________ Increased lordotic curve: ____________________

ACTIVE CERVICAL RANGE OF MOTION:

Flexion (45° - 55°)		________	P	Extension (70°)		________	P
Rotation (80° - 85°)	R	________	P	Lateroflexion (45°)	R	________	P
	L	________	P		L	________	P

Comments: ____________________

____

PASSIVE CERVICAL MOBILITY: ____________________

ACTIVE UPPER EXTREMITY RANGE OF MOTION:

Shoulder Flexion (160° - 180°)	R	________	P	Shoulder Abduction (120°)	R	________	P
	L	________	P		L	________	P

Comments: ____________________

____

RESISTED CERVICAL MOTIONS:

Flexion		________	P	Extension		________	P
Rotation	R	________	P	Lateroflexion	R	________	P
	L	________	P		L	________	P

KEY
1 = Trace
2 = Poor
3 = Fair
4 = Good
5 = Normal

UPPER EXTREMITY STRENGTH:

Shoulder Flexion	R	________	P	Shoulder Abduction	R	________	P
	L	________	P		L	________	P
Scapular Muscles	R	________	P				
	L	________	P				

Number of shoulder shrugs: ________

Comments: ____________________

____

TENDERNESS TO PALPATION:

Sternocleidomastoid	R ________	L ________	Trapezius	R ________	L ________
Scaleni	R ________	L ________	Suboccipitals	R ________	L ________
Levator Scapula	R ________	L ________	Rhomboids	R ________	L ________

-2-

TMJ EVALUATION

Patient Name ____________________

Patient Number ____________________

TENDERNESS TO PALPATION:

Masseter	R ________	L ________
Temporalis	R ________	L ________
Medial Pterygoid	R ________	L ________
TMJ Lateral Pole	R ________	L ________

Comments: ____

____

MECHANICS:

Maximum opening: ________ mm [P]

Mouth opening/closing deviation (mm)

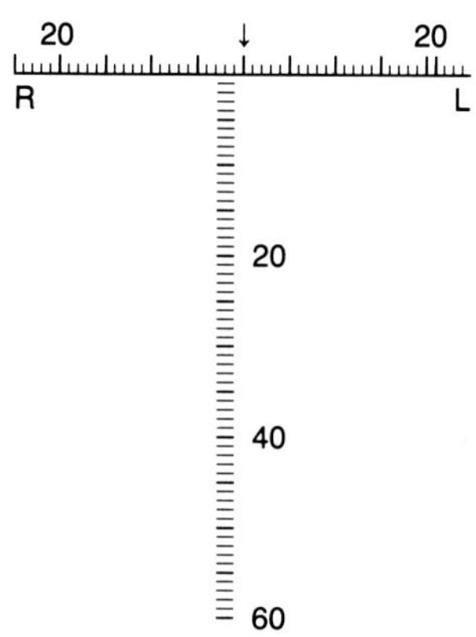

Deviation:	☐ Yes	☐ No	Right	P	Left	P
Deflection:	☐ Yes	☐ No	Right	P	Left	P
Joint Noises:	☐ Yes	☐ No	Right	P	Left	P

Describe: ____________________________

Where: ____________________________

Protrusion:	________ mm	P
Left laterotrusion:	________ mm	P
Right laterotrusion:	________ mm	P

OVERALL JOINT MOBILITY:

1 = hypomobile 2 = normal 3 = hypermobile

JOINT PLAY:

Distraction:	Right	P	Left	P
Translation:	Right	P	Left	P

Retrusive overpressure: Right ________ [P] Left ________ [P]

OTHER: ____

____

____

____

____

Changes noted/reported when posture was corrected: ______

Clinical impression/assessment: ______

Problem List	Short Term Goals	Long Term Goals

Treatment Plan: ______

Preliminary diagnosis from the referring doctor: ______

SIGNATURE ______ DATE ______

-4-

References

Agerberg G (1974): Maximal mandibular movements in young men and women. *Swed Dent J* 67:81–100.

Antoniotti T, Rocabado M (1990): *Exercise and Total Well-Being for Vertebral and Craniomandibular Disorders.* Tucson, IFORC Publications.

Bezuur JN, Habets LLMH, Jimenez Lopez V, Naeije M, Hansson TL (1988a): The recognition of craniomandibular disorders—a comparison between clinical and radiographic findings in eighty-nine subjects. *J Oral Rehabil* 15:215–221.

Bezuur JN, Habets LLMH, Hansson TL (1988b): The recognition of craniomandibular disorders—a comparison between clinical, tomographical, and dental panoramic radiographical findings in thirty-one subjects. *J Oral Rehabil* 15:549–554.

Bezuur JN, Habets LLMH, Hansson TL (1988c): The effect of therapeutic laser treatment in patients with craniomandibular disorders. *J Craniomandib Disord Facial Oral Pain* 2:83–86.

Bezuur JN, Habets LLMH, Hansson TL (1989a): The recognition of craniomandibular disorders: condylar symmetry in relation to myogenous and arthrogenous origin of pain. *J Oral Rehabil* 16:257–260.

Bezuur JN, Hansson TL, Wilkinson TM (1989b): The recognition of craniomandibular disorders—an evaluation of the most reliable signs and symptoms when screening for CMD. *J Oral Rehabil* 16:367–372.

Hansson TL (1989): Infrared laser in the treatment of craniomandibular disorders, arthrogenous pain. *J Prosthet Dent* 61:614–617.

Hansson TL (1990): Progress report sull'impiego del laser a raggi infrarossi nel trattamentto del dolore nelle disfunzioni temporomandibolari su base artrogena. *G Odontol Gnatol* 5:11–13.

Hansson T, Wessman C, Oberg T (1980): Säkrare diagnoser med ny teknik. Förslag till funktionsbedömningar av käkleder och tuggmuskler. *Tandläkartidningen* 72:1372–1374.

Hansson T, Honee W, Hesse J (1985): *Craniomandibulaire Dysfunctie.* Alphen aan den Rijn/Brussel, Samsom Stafleu.

Janda V (1976): Muskelfunktionsdiagnostik. Lund, Student Litteratur.

Kaltenborn E (1974): *Manual Therapy for Extremity Joints.* Oslo, Forlag Olaf Norlins Boghandel.

Kraus SL (1988): *TMJ Disorders, Management of the Craniomandibular Complex.* New York, Edinburgh, London, Melbourne, Churchill Livingstone.

Naeije M, Hansson, TL (1986): Electromyographic screening of myogenous and arthrogenous TMJ dysfunction patients. *J Oral Rehabil* 13:433–441.

Schokker RP, Hansson TL, Ansink BJJ (1989): Craniomandibular disorders in headache patients. *J Craniomandib Disord Facial Oral Pain* 3:71–74.

Schokker RP, Hansson TL, Ansink BJJ (1990a): Craniomandibular disorders in patients with different types of headache. *J Craniomandib Disord Facial Oral Pain* 4:47–51.

Schokker RP, Hansson TL, Ansink BJJ (1990b): Differences in headache patients regarding response to treatment of the masticatory system. *J Craniomandib Disord Facial Oral Pain* 4:228–232.